An Aid to
RESPIRATORY MEDICINE
for Postgraduate Exit Exam

MD, DNB and Diploma

An Aid to
RESPIRATORY MEDICINE
for Postgraduate Exit Exam

MD, DNB and Diploma

Editor

Susmita Kundu

MBBS DTM&H MD(TB and Chest Diseases) DNB(RPD)
Professor and Head
Department of Respiratory Medicine
KPC Medical College
Ex-Professor and Head
Department of Respiratory Medicine
RG Kar Medical College and Hospital
Kolkata, West Bengal, India

Foreword

Digambar Behera

(Padma Awardee)

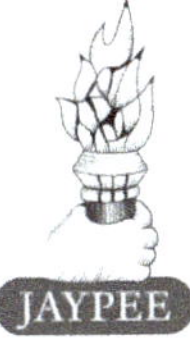

JAYPEE BROTHERS MEDICAL PUBLISHERS
The Health Sciences Publisher
New Delhi | London

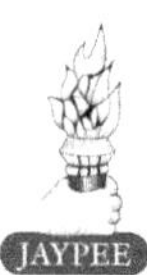 **Jaypee Brothers Medical Publishers (P) Ltd**

Headquarters
EMCA House
23/23-B, Ansari Road, Daryaganj
New Delhi 110 002, India
Landline: +91-11-23272143, +91-11-23272703
+91-11-23282021, +91-11-23245672
E-mail: jaypee@jaypeebrothers.com

Corporate Office
Jaypee Brothers Medical Publishers (P) Ltd.
4838/24, Ansari Road, Daryaganj
New Delhi 110 002, India
Phone: +91-11-43574357
Fax: +91-11-43574314
E-mail: jaypee@jaypeebrothers.com

Overseas Office
JP Medical Ltd.
83, Victoria Street, London
SW1H 0HW (UK)
Phone: +44-20 3170 8910
E-mail: info@jpmedpub.com

EU GPSR Authorised Representative
Logos Europe, 9 rue Nicolas Poussin
17000, La Rochelle, France
Phone: +33 (0) 6 67 93 73 78
E-mail: Contact@logoseurope.eu

Website: www.jaypeebrothers.com
Website: www.jaypeedigital.com

© 2025, Jaypee Brothers Medical Publishers

Inquiries for bulk sales may be solicited at: jaypee@jaypeebrothers.com

An Aid to Respiratory Medicine for Postgraduate Exit Exam (MD, DNB and Diploma) / Susmita Kundu

First Edition: 2025

ISBN: 978-93-5696-937-7

Contributors

Arya Chaudhuri MBBS MD(Respiratory Medicine)
Senior Resident
Department of Respiratory Medicine
RG Kar Medical College and Hospital
Kolkata, West Bengal, India

Saikat Banerjee MBBS MD(Respiratory Medicine) DM(Pulmonary, Critical Care and
Sleep Medicine)
Senior Resident
Department of Respiratory Medicine
College of Medicine and Sagore Dutta Hospital
Kolkata, West Bengal, India

Susmita Kundu MBBS DTM&H MD(TB and Chest Diseases) DNB(RPD)
Professor and Head
Department of Respiratory Medicine
KPC Medical College
Ex-Professor and Head
Department of Respiratory Medicine
RG Kar Medical College and Hospital
Kolkata, West Bengal, India

Foreword

The book entitled *"An Aid to Respiratory Medicine for Postgraduate Exit Exam (MD, DNB and Diploma)"* is a timely and an appropriate guide for students for their exit examination. It will be a good help for all those who aspire for success in the subject. The author of the book Professor (Dr) Susmita Kundu is presently the Head of Department of Respiratory Medicine, RG Kar Medical College and Hospital, Kolkata, West Bengal, India. She is very well known in the field of pulmonary (respiratory) medicine in the country and an excellent teacher. Professor Kundu carries with her vast experience in the field of respiratory medicine in India. A clinician, researcher, and teacher par excellence, Dr Kundu has given very good inputs and guidance to the students through this book. It will be a very useful addition in the field of respiratory medicine and of very much help to the students and practitioners in the field. The book has six chapters with illustrated chest X-rays, CT thorax, USG thorax, pulmonary function test, arterial blood gas (ABG), and polysomnography. All chapters are independent and can be read separately.

I congratulate Dr Kundu for this piece of useful work and I hope that an innumerable number of our young colleagues will benefit from this. I wish all success for the book brought out by Dr Susmita out of her years of rich experience.

Digambar Behera

Digambar Behera
(Padma Awardee)
MD(Medicine) FCCP FAMS FNCCP FICP FICA FAPSR FICS
MNAMS(Medicine) Dip NBE(Respiratory Medicine)
Emeritus Professor and Former Professor and Head
Department of Pulmonary Medicine (WHO Collaborating Centre for Research and
Capacity Building in Chronic Respiratory Diseases)
Ex-Dean (Research), Ex-Chairman of Medical Departments (Group B)
Postgraduate Institute of Medical Education and Research, Chandigarh
Advisor, National Task Force (NTEP/RNTCP)
President, Indian Society for Study of Lung Cancer
President-Elect, National Academy of Medical Sciences
Past-President, National College of Chest Physicians
Ex-President, Indian Chest Society
EX-OSD, AIIMS, Raebareli, Uttar Pradesh
Director, Pulmonary Medicine, Fortis Health Care, Mohali (Currently)

Preface

Collection of interesting chest X-rays, CT scans of thorax, USG thorax, pulmonary function test reports, and arterial blood gas analysis charts is a very good academic hobby for a pulmonologist. It immensely helps to teach students, both undergraduate and postgraduate, as well as those who are taking final examination at all levels. Findings of chest X-ray with differential diagnosis and most probable diagnosis as well as CT scans of thorax will help students as well as practitioners to think about the cause and proceed further to clinch the final diagnosis. Likewise, pulmonary function results will differentiate between obstructive and restrictive or combined disease and will justify the treatment for better patient care. Analysis of bedside blood gas reports will save many lives.

In the modern era, knowing about sleep disorders and their management will improve the skill and quality of life of many sufferers.

We hope that this book will help our students as well as practitioners and ultimately provide valuable information and knowledge to help the patients.

Susmita Kundu

Acknowledgments

The work done in this book has been brought to fruition through the efforts, ideas, thoughts, and invaluable time of many, all of whom I want to acknowledge.

It is my best and proud privilege to express my deep sense of gratitude to my colleague, Professor (Dr) Jayatee Bardhan, Professor and Head, Department of Radiodiagnosis, RG Kar Medical College and Hospital, West Bengal, Kolkata, India. I am indebted to her from the very first step of this process. Her zealous involvement, keen interest, and valuable suggestions at every step of my work set an example for me to follow.

I felicitate my sincere thanks to Dr Debasish Karmakar, RMO, Department of Respiratory Medicine, RG Kar Medical College and Hospital, for his invaluable support and contribution.

I would also like to thank all the faculties and students of Department of Respiratory Medicine, RG Kar Medical College and Hospital, including the postgraduate trainees of my unit for their unwavering support and contribution, without which this book would not have been possible.

I am also obliged to Professor (Dr) Atin Dey, Mr Jayanta De and Mr Atanu Bhattacharya for their help and contribution.

I am deeply grateful to Shri Jitendar P Vij (Group Chairman), Mr Ankit Vij (Managing Director), Mr MS Mani (Group President), Ms Chetna Malhotra (Senior Director—Professional Publishing, Marketing, and Business Development), Ms Pooja Bhandari [Director—Production (Books and Journals)], and Mr Akhilesh Saxena (Publishing Coordinator), M/s Jaypee Brothers Medical Publishers (P) Ltd, New Delhi, India, for their professional support and dedication to bringing this book to life. Their team has been phenomenal for being there for me round the clock with their platform and commitment to enhancing and propagating scientific learning and knowledge.

Lastly, I would like to express my gratitude to Mr Abhishek Banerjee and Mr Sabyasachi Nayak for clicking such wonderful pictures for this book.

Thanks to the Almighty!

Susmita Kundu

Contents

Chest X-ray

Susmita Kundu

INTRODUCTION

- The chest X-ray (CXR) remains one of the most commonly ordered imaging studies in chest medicine in spite of many advancement in chest imaging, because of its low cost and single source.
- Chest X-ray produces images of the heart, lungs, blood vessels, airways, and the bones of chest and spine.
- It can also reveal fluid in or around the lungs or air surrounding a lung.
- It is often also the most difficult investigation to interpret.

X-RAY ABSORPTION AND PENETRATION

- X-ray absorption and penetration (transmission) are the reciprocal of each other.
- The differential absorption of radiation by different tissues or diseases is responsible for all radiographic images. Air, fat, soft tissue (muscle, fluid), and metal (bone) absorb progressively more radiation. The thicker the tissue, the more it absorbs.
- Fat appears gray or less radiolucent than air, and soft tissue appears white with slight radiopacity.
- Bone absorbs more radiation so bone is said to be radiodense, because radiation hardly penetrate it.

CHEST RADIOLOGY

- Patient to machine distance 6 feet
- Observer to X-ray distance 3 feet
- To be taken in full inspiration
- Ray from behind and patient in front—in posteroanterior (PA) view **(Figs. 1 and 2)**

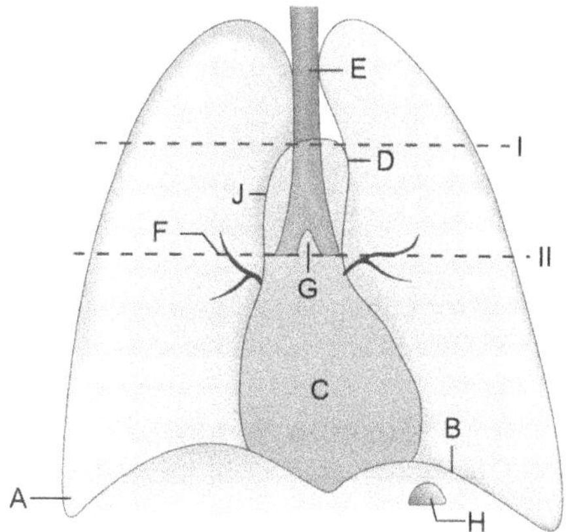

FIG. 1: Landmarks in normal chest X-ray posteroanterior (PA) view.

Note: A—costophrenic angle, B—left diaphragm, C—heart, D—aortic arch, E—trachea, F—hilum, G—carina, H—stomach bubble, J—ascending aorta.

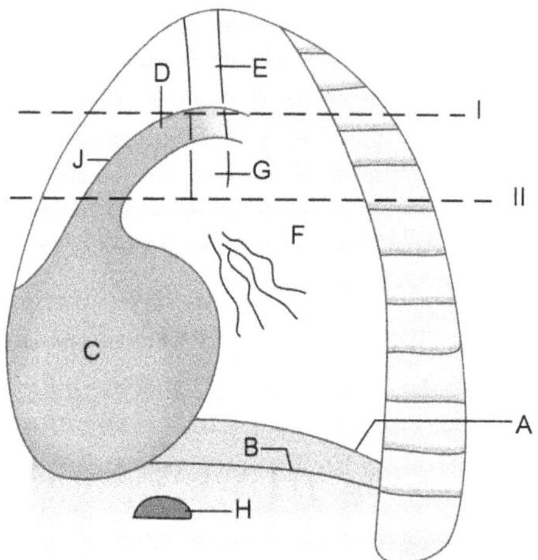

FIG. 2: Landmarks in normal chest X-ray lateral view.

Note: A—costophrenic angle, B—left diaphragm, C—heart, D—aortic arch, E—trachea, F—hilum, G—carina, H—stomach bubble, J—ascending aorta.

FELSON'S PRINCIPLES OF CHEST ROENTGENOLOGY (FIGS. 3A AND B)

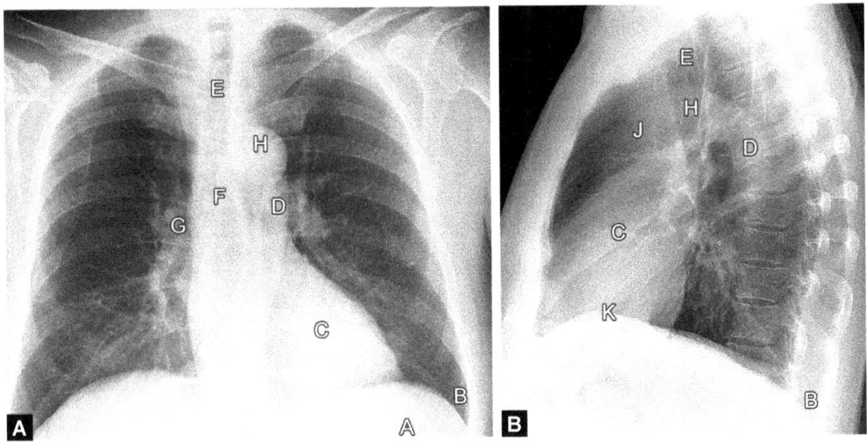

FIGS. 3A AND B: Principles of chest roentgenology.

Note: A—gas in splenic flexure, B—costophrenic angle, C—heart, D—descending aorta, E—trachea, F—carina, G—hilum, H—aortic knob, J—ascending aorta, K—right diaphragm.

WHAT YOU LOOK FOR IN APPARENT NORMAL CHEST X-RAY?

- Cervical rib
- Azygos lobe
- Left lower lobe collapse
- Mastectomy
- Rib erosion
- Subpulmonic effusion

INCREASED CARDIAC SILHOUETTE

- Diameter of heart >50% of transthoracic diameter
- Any heart larger than 15.5 cm is probably pathologically enlarged heart
- A difference of >1.5 cm from previous CXR

CHEST X-RAY 1

- *Description*: Homogeneous opacity occupying left, mid, and lower zone, curved upper border and heart shifted toward right side.
- *Differential diagnosis*:
  - Massive left sided pleural effusion
  - Left side lung mass with pleural effusion
  - Pleural mesothelioma—left
- *Final impression*: Left sided massive pleural effusion

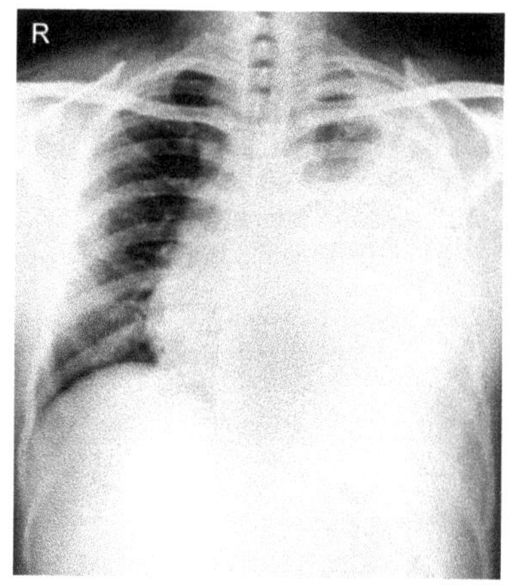

CHEST X-RAY 2

- *Description*: Right sided increased translucency and absence of bronchovascular marking with complete collapse of right lung.
- *Differential diagnosis*:
  - Right sided complete pneumothorax
  - Right sided MacLeod syndrome
- *Final impression*: Right sided complete pneumothorax

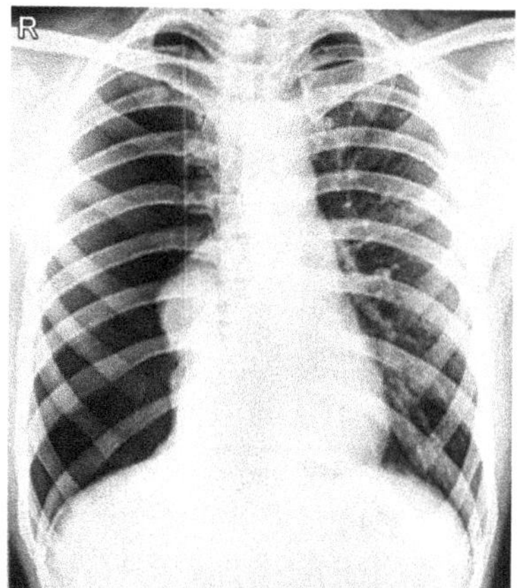

CHEST X-RAY 3

- *Description*: Right sided increased translucency with air fluid level
- *Final impression*: Right sided hydropneumothorax

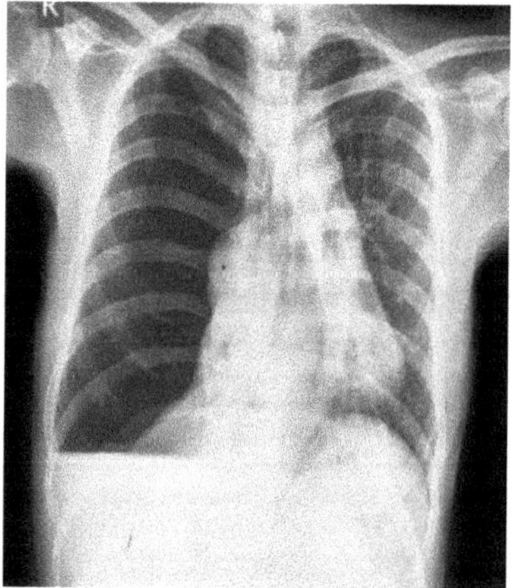

CHEST X-RAY 4

- *Description*: Increased cardiac silhouette with right sided pleural effusion with thickening of transverse fissure.
- *Differential diagnosis*:
  - Mild pericardial effusion with right sided pleural effusion
  - Heart failure [e.g., ischemic heart disease (IHD), valvular heart disease, and cardiomyopathy]
  - Severe anemia with heart failure
- *Final impression*: Heart failure

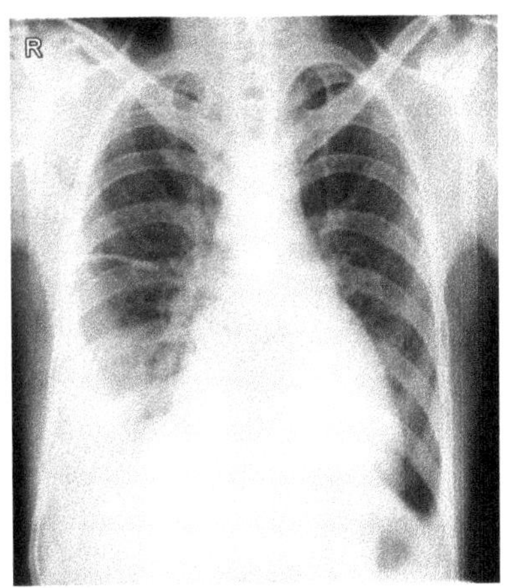

CHEST X-RAY 5

- *Description*: Right sided homogeneous opacity seen in right lower and mid part, and denser opacity with sharp margin with base toward pleura seen in right mid zone.
- *Impression*: Right sided pleural effusion with right costal encystment—D sign.

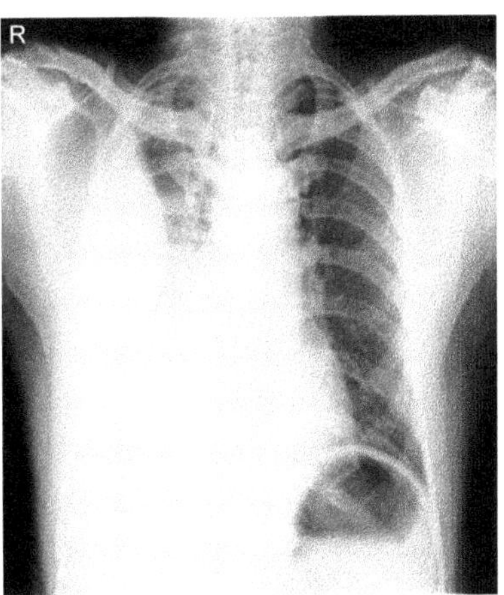

CHEST X-RAY 6

- *Description*: Left upper zone D-shaped homogeneous opacity with base toward pleura with left mid zone lung abscess with left lower cardiophrenic angle obliterated.
- *Final impression*: Left sided pneumonia with lung abscess and encysted pleural effusion.

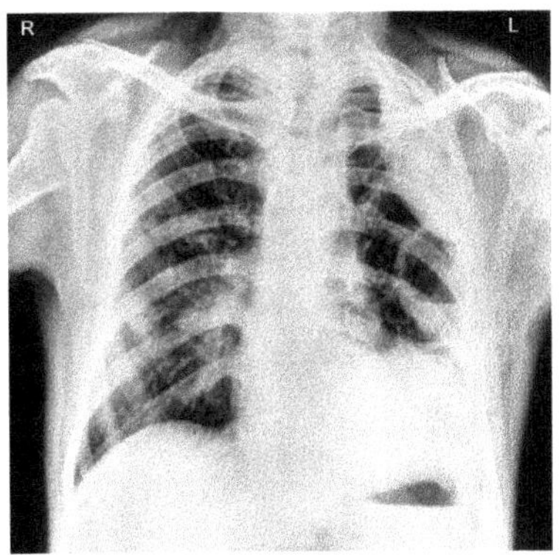

CHEST X-RAY 7

- *Description*: Right sided peripherally located nonhomogeneous dense calcified opacity with obliteration of right costophrenic (CP) angle.
- *Differential diagnosis*:
  - Pleural calcification following empyema
  - Asbestos related benign pleural calcification
- *Final impression*: Pleural calcification—sequelae of empyema

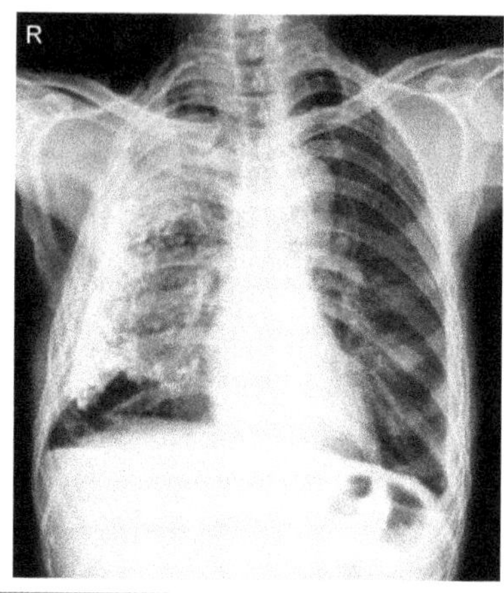

CHEST X-RAY 8

- *Description*: Bilateral pleural thickening with calcification right > left (r > l)—molten candle wax
- *Differential diagnosis*:
  - Bilateral asbestos related benign pleural calcification
  - Bilateral postempyema pleural calcification
- *Final impression*: Bilateral postempyema calcification

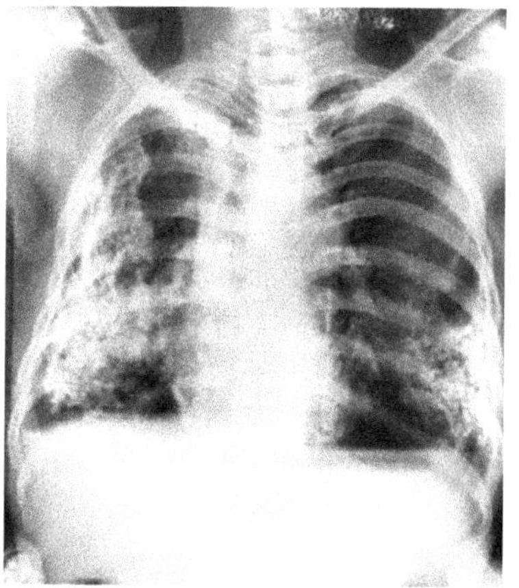

CHEST X-RAY 9

- *Description*: Right upper and mid zone homogeneous opacity with air bronchogram with bulging of transverse fissure.
- *Final impression*: Right upper lobe pneumonia with bulging fissure sign classically seen in *Klebsiella pneumonia*.

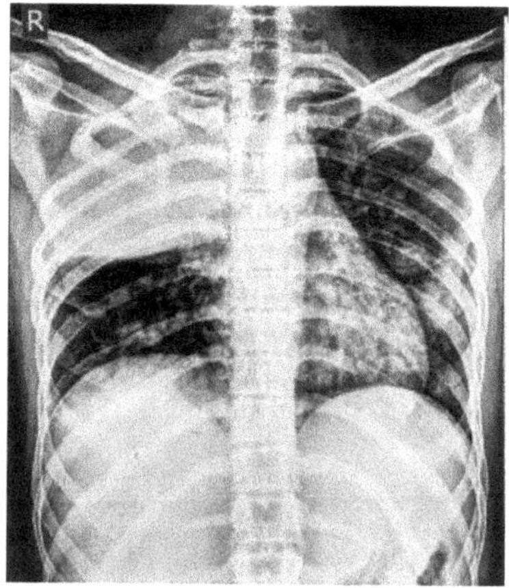

CHEST X-RAY 10

- *Description*: Right mid and lower zone cavitary lesion with air fluid level with clear right CP angle.
- *Differential diagnosis*:
  - Right sided lung abscess
  - Right sided encysted hydropneumothorax
  - Right sided ruptured hydatid cyst
  - Right sided infected bullae
- *Final impression*: Right sided lung abscess

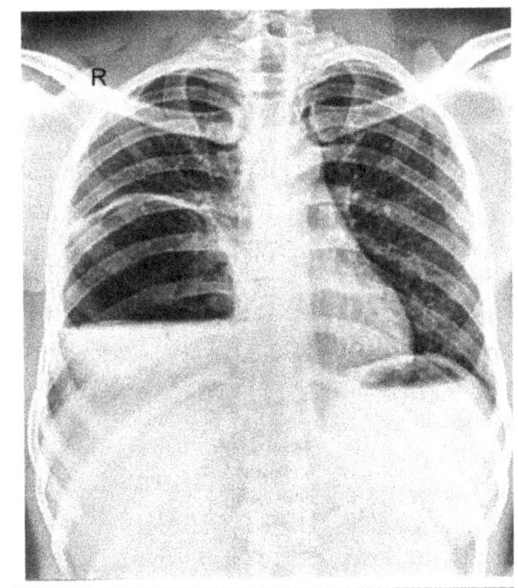

CHEST X-RAY 11

- *Description*: Bilateral extensive micronodular shadows with small cavity in right upper zone.
- *Differential diagnosis*:
  - Tuberculosis (TB)
  - Secondary deposits from distal organ malignancy
  - Occupational lung disease
  - Tropical pulmonary eosinophilia
  - Primary lung malignancy
  - Fungal disease
- *Final impression*: TB

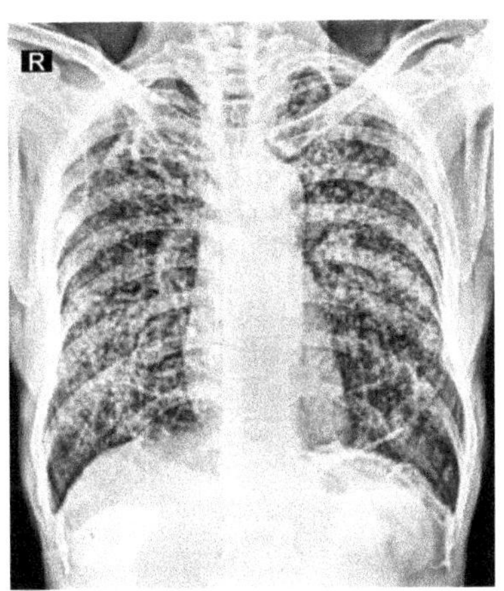

CHEST X-RAY 12

- *Description*: Bilateral extensive miliary opacities with left sided minimal pleural effusion.
- *Differential diagnosis*:
  - Miliary TB with left sided minimal pleural effusion
  - Secondary deposits with left sided minimal pleural effusion
  - Pneumoconiosis/Silicosis
  - Bacterial infection (staph)
  - Fungal infection
  - Tropical pulmonary eosinophilia
- *Final impression*: Miliary TB

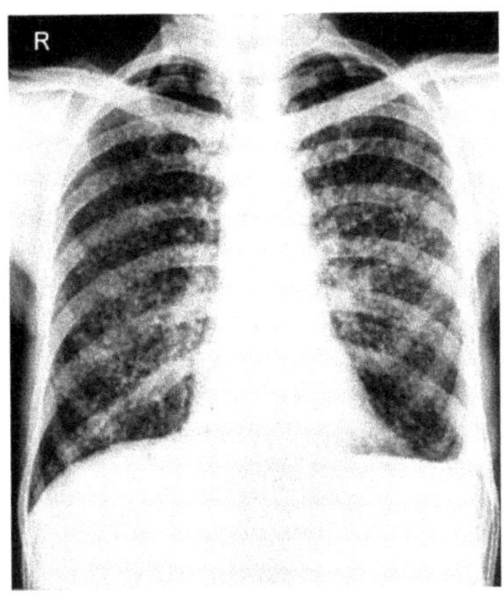

CHEST X-RAY 13

- *Description*: Bilateral multiple nodular opacities with coalescence predominantly in the left lower zone with right sided mastectomy.
- *Differential diagnosis*:
  - Mastectomy in a case of right sided breast cancer (CA) with bilateral pulmonary metastasis
  - Mastectomy in a case of right sided breast CA with bacterial infection
  - Mastectomy in a case of right sided breast CA with fungal infection
  - Mastectomy in a case of right sided breast CA with TB
- *Final impression*: Mastectomy in a case of right sided breast CA with bilateral pulmonary metastasis

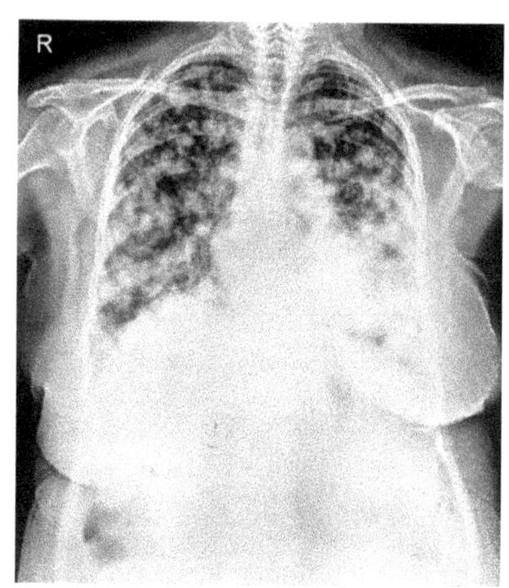

CHEST X-RAY 14

- *Description*: Bilateral extensive nodular opacities
- *Differential diagnosis*:
  - Secondary metastasis
  - TB
  - Fungal infection
  - Pneumonia
- *Final impression*: Secondary metastasis

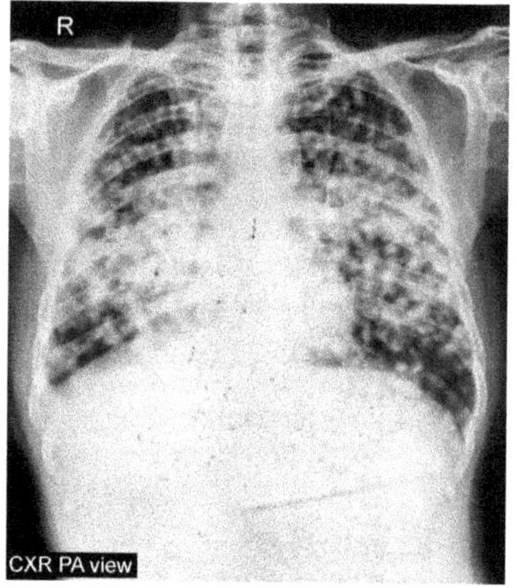

CHEST X-RAY 15

- *Description*: Bilateral extensive nodular opacities
- *Differential diagnosis*:
  - TB
  - Bacterial pneumonia
  - Fungal disease
  - Primary lung malignancy with secondary metastasis
  - Lung metastasis
  - Sarcoid
- *Final impression*: Lung metastasis

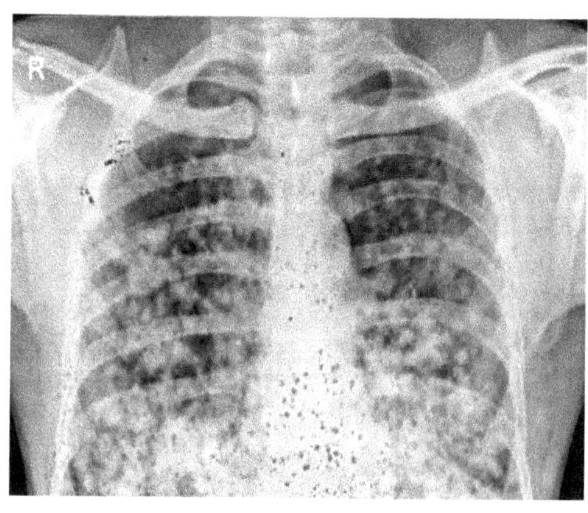

CHEST X-RAY 16

- *Description*: Bilateral extensive fibrocavitory lesion with air-fluid level in one cavity in left mid zone with obliteration of left CP angle.
- *Differential diagnosis*:
  - Bilateral cystic bronchiectasis with infection
  - Bilateral extensive post TB sequelae
- *Final impression*: Bilateral cystic bronchiectasis with one infected cavity in left mid zone with minimal pleural effusion left.

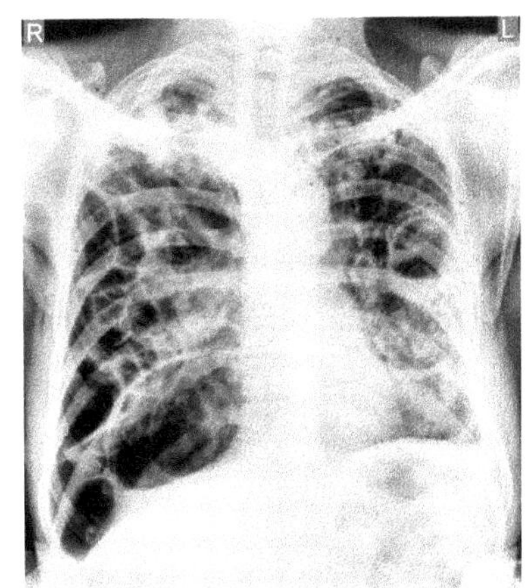

CHEST X-RAY 17

- *Description*: Right mid zone intracavitary body with air crescent sign (meniscus sign)
- *Differential diagnosis*:
  - Aspergilloma right lung
  - Intracavitary mass
  - Intracavitary blood clot
- *Final impression*: Right sided aspergilloma

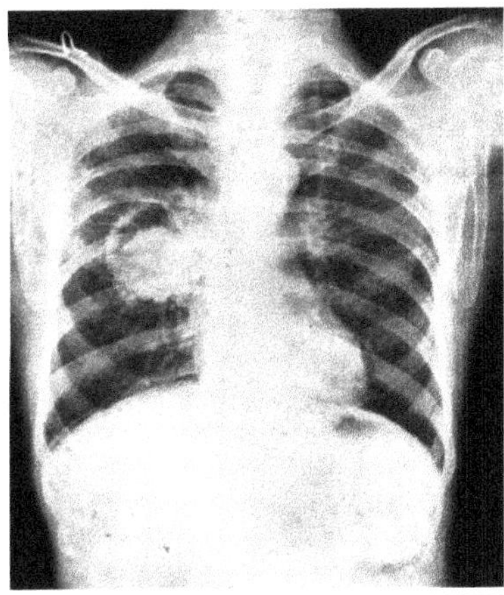

CHEST X-RAY 18

- *Description*: Left sided lung abscess with right sided multiple cavities.
- *Differential diagnosis*:
  - Multiple pneumatocele following staphylococcal pneumonia
  - *Klebsiella pneumoniae*
  - Multiple infected bullae
  - TB
- *Final impression*: Multiple pneumatocele following staphylococcal pneumonia.

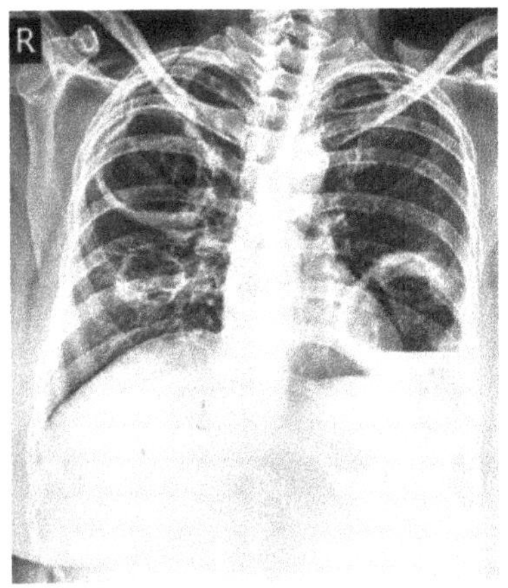

CHEST X-RAY 19

- *Description*: Bilateral extensive opacity sparing both upper part and left lower part.
- *Differential diagnosis*:
  - Chronic eosinophilic pneumonia (CEP)
  - Acute interstitial pneumonia (AIP)
  - Acute eosinophilic pneumonia
  - Acute respiratory distress syndrome (ARDS)
  - Pulmonary edema
  - *Pneumocystis jerovecii* pneumonia (PJP)

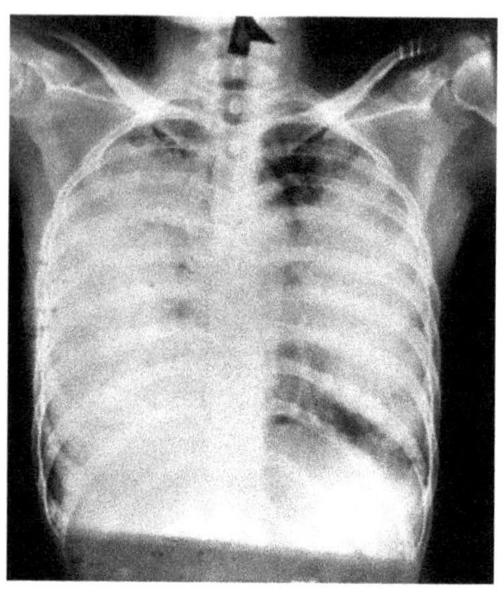

CHEST X-RAY 20

- *Description*: Bilateral mid and lower zone nonhomogeneous opacity sparing both CP angles and blurring of both heart borders.
- *Differential diagnosis*:
  - Pulmonary edema
  - PJP
  - ARDS
  - AIP
- *Final impression*: Pulmonary edema

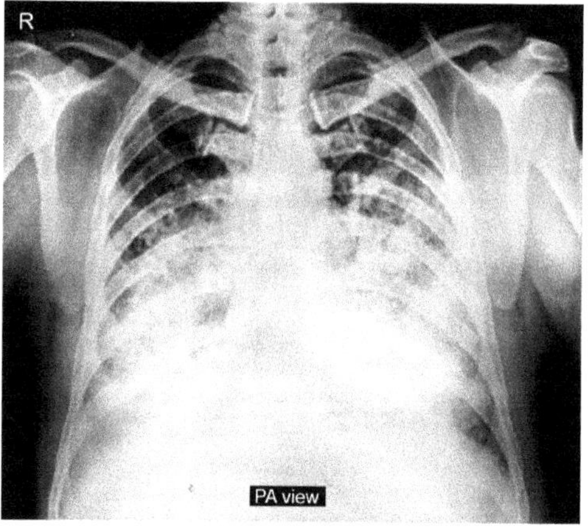

CHEST X-RAY 21

- Bilateral peripheral nonhomogeneous opacity sparing the apical regions and paracardiac areas.
- *Differential diagnosis*:
  - Bilateral pneumonia
  - CEP
  - Organizing pneumonia
  - AIP
  - Secondary metastasis
- *Final impression*: Secondary metastasis (biopsy proven)

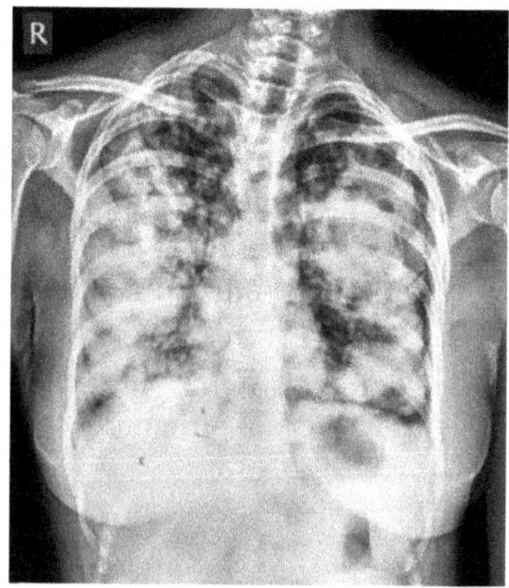

CHEST X-RAY 22

- *Description*: Bilateral pneumothorax with right sided implantable cardioverter defibrillator (ICD) in situ with bilateral mid zone homogeneous dense opacity (r > l), with bilateral multiple nodular opacities in both lower zone.
- *Differential diagnosis*:
  - Bilateral progressive massive fibrosis (PMF) in silicosis/coal worker's pneumoconiosis (CWP) with bilateral pneumothorax with right sided ICD in situ.
  - Predominantly bilateral extensive TB with bilateral pneumothorax with right sided ICD in situ.
- *Final impression*: Bilateral pneumothorax in a case of silicosis with PMF with right sided ICD in situ.

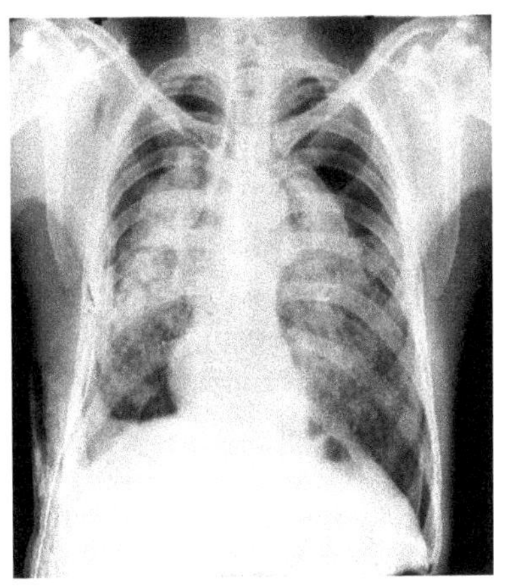

CHEST X-RAY 23

- *Description*: Bilateral upper and mid zone reticulo-nodular opacities
- *Differential diagnosis*:
  - Hypersensitivity pneumonitis
  - TB
  - Silicosis
  - Pulmonary Langerhans cell histiocytosis
- *Final impression*: Hypersensitivity pneumonitis

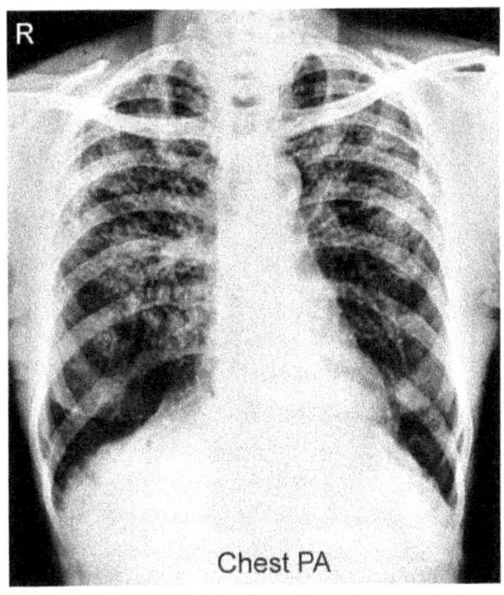

CHEST X-RAY 24

- *Description*: Black hyper lucency seen in left side with shifting of mediastinum toward opposite side (orientation is not proper)
- *Differential diagnosis*:
  - Left sided pneumothorax
  - Left sided giant bulla
- *Final impression*: Left sided giant bulla (as no collapse lung present)

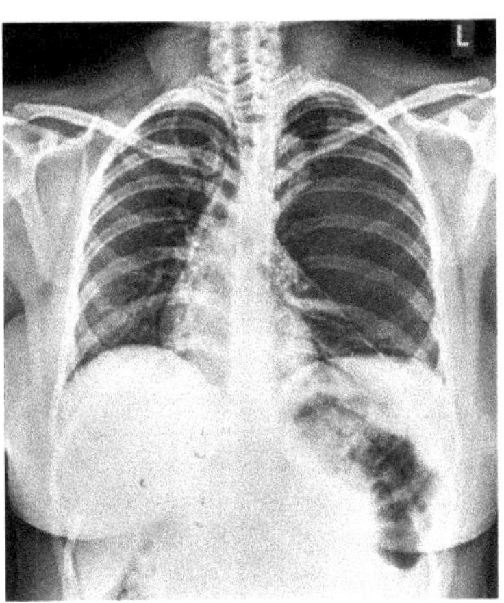

CHEST X-RAY 25

- *Description*: Well-defined dense homogeneous opacity with smooth well circumscribed margin in right mid zone.
- *Differential diagnosis*:
  - Hydatid cyst
  - Lung abscess (before rupture)
  - Mediastinal tumor
  - Bronchogenic cyst
- *Final impression*: Mediastinal tumor

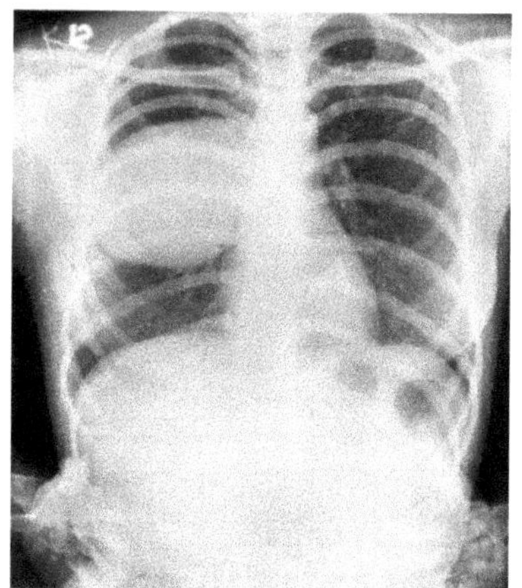

CHEST X-RAY 26

- *Description*: Left hilar opacity with well-defined lower margin and sun ray burst sign in the upper part.
- *Differential diagnosis*:
  - Sun ray burst appearance in a case of left hilar mass (malignant)
  - Left mid zone consolidation (parahilar)
- *Final impression*: Left hilar mass (malignant)

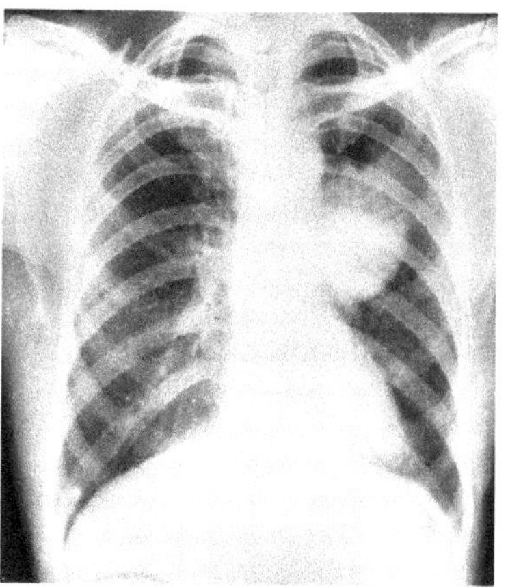

CHEST X-RAY 27

- *Description*: Nonhomogeneous opacity in right upper zone with smooth lower margin and more opaque medial side of the opacity.
- *Differential diagnosis*:
  - Hamartoma
  - Schwannoma
- *Final impression*: Schwannoma-biopsy proven

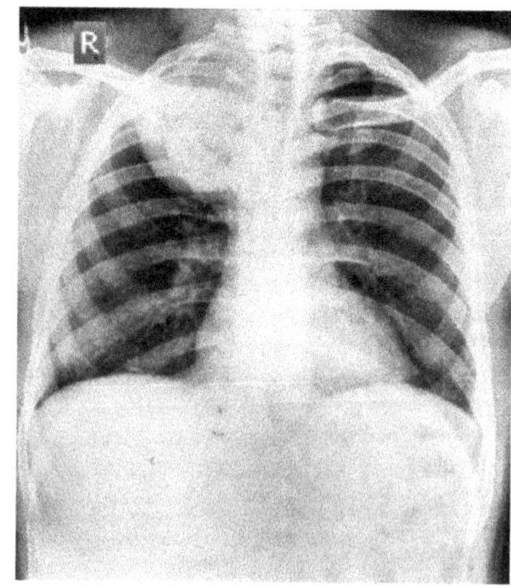

CHEST X-RAY 28

- *Description*: Lower mid zone and lower zone homogeneous opacity with well-defined margin obscuring left heart border.
- *Differential diagnosis*:
  - Lingular mass
  - Pneumonia in lingular region
  - Left ventricular aneurysm
- *Final impression*: After lateral CXR—lingular mass

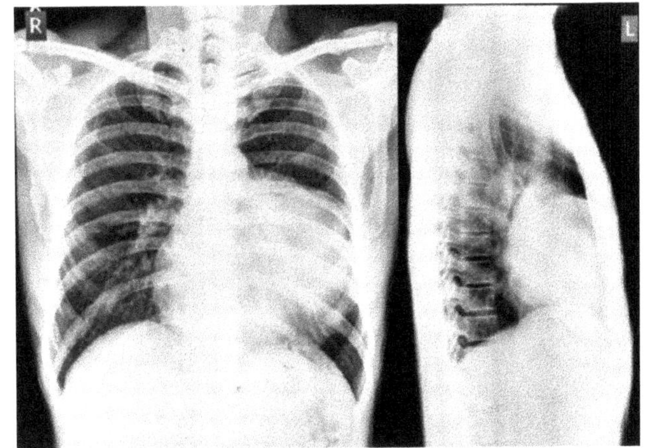

CHEST X-RAY 29

- *Description*: Right mid and lower zone homogeneous opacity with sharp margin predominantly in the lower part.
- *Differential diagnosis*:
  - Right lung space occupying lesion (SOL)
  - Right sided pneumonia without cardiac silhouette
  - Right lung hydatid cyst
- *Final impression*: Right lung SOL

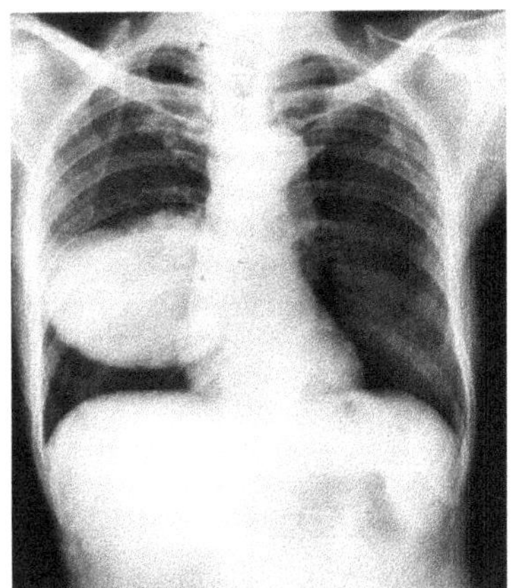

CHEST X-RAY 30

- *Description*: Big round opacity left mid and lower zone with well-defined heart border.
- *Differential diagnosis*:
  - Hydatid cyst
  - Left lung SOL
  - Lung abscess before rupture
  - Mediastinal mass
- *Final impression*: Hydatid cyst

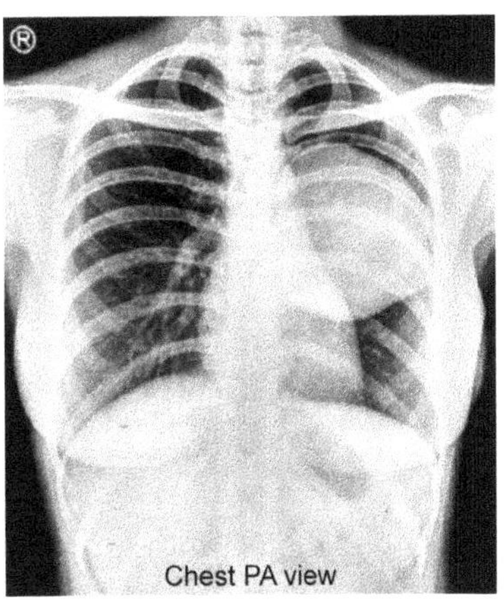

Chest PA view

CHEST X-RAY 31

- *Description*: Well-defined round opacities—one on right side and two on left side.
- *Differential diagnosis*:
  - Multiple hydatid cyst
  - Multiple lung abscess
  - Multiple canon ball shadows
- *Final impression*: Multiple hydatid cyst

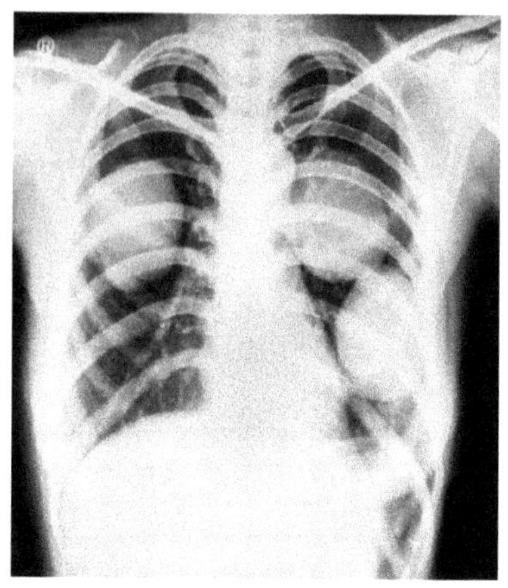

CHEST X-RAY 32

- *Description*: Multiple homogeneous well-defined opacities of varying sizes in both lung fields.
- *Differential diagnosis*:
  - Multiple hydatid cyst
  - Multiple neurofibroma
- *Final impression*: Multiple hydatid cyst in both lung

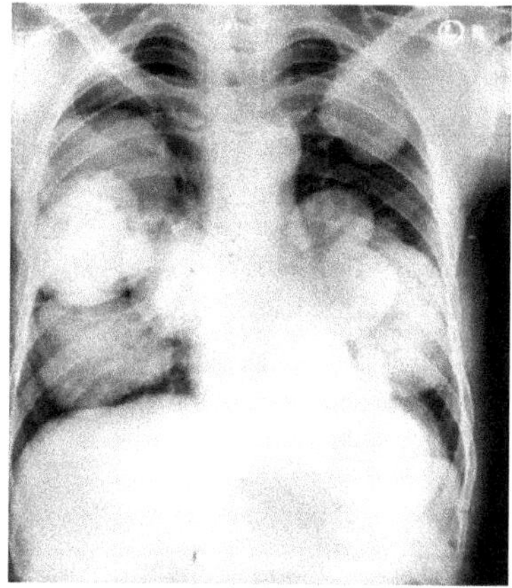

CHEST X-RAY 33

- *Description*: Homogeneous opacity in left lower zone with upward shifting of left hemidiaphragm with shifting of trachea to left side with left lung volume loss.
- *Differential diagnosis*:
  - Left destroyed lung
  - Left lower lobe collapse of some duration
  - Left lower lobectomy
- *Final impression*: Left lower lobe collapse of some duration.

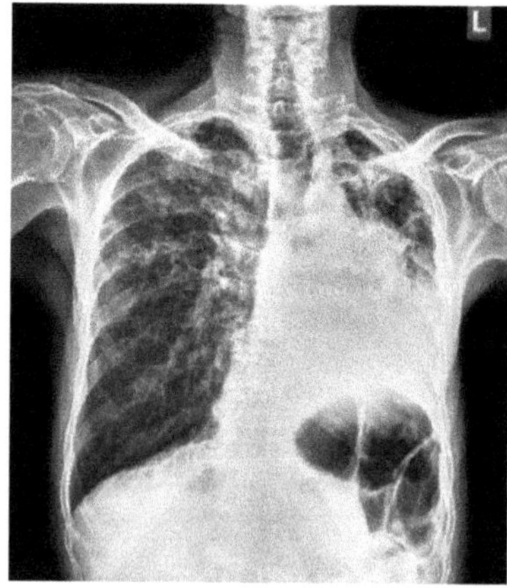

CHEST X-RAY 34

- *Description*: Shifting of heart toward left with bilateral diaphragm at same level, with homogeneous opacity in left upper zone sparing left CP angle, and sickle-shaped shadow in left paratracheal area and beside the aortic knuckle.
- *Impression:* Luftsichel sign—luftsichel is a German word meaning air crescent (luft—air, sichel—sickel). This sign is seen in some cases of left upper lobe collapse and refers to the frontal chest radiographic appearance due to hyperinflation of the superior segment of left lower lobe interposing itself between aortic arch, mediastinum, and the collapsed left upper lobe.

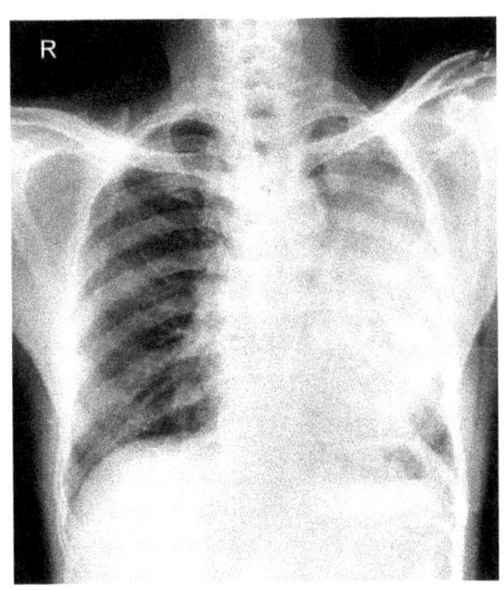

CHEST X-RAY 35

- Double left heart border with elevation of left hemidiaphragm.
- *Final impression*: Left lower lobe collapse.

Note: Left lower lobe collapse should always be looked for in an apparently normal CXR.

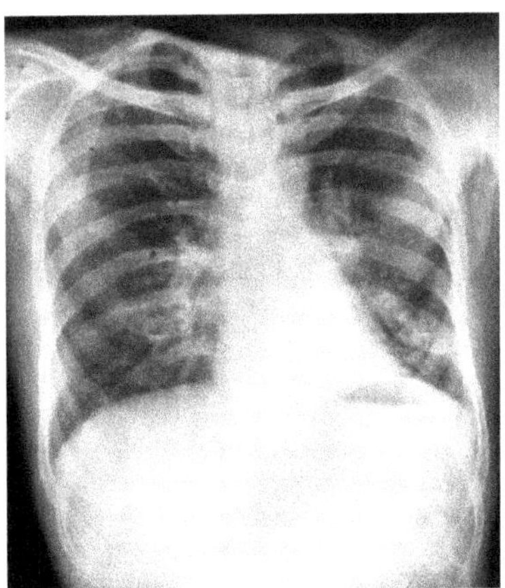

CHEST X-RAY 36

- Triangular opacity in right lower zone paracardiac area with diaphragmatic silhouette.
- *Differential diagnosis*:
  - Right lower lobe collapse
  - Pericardial pad of fat
- *Final impression*: Right lower lobe collapse

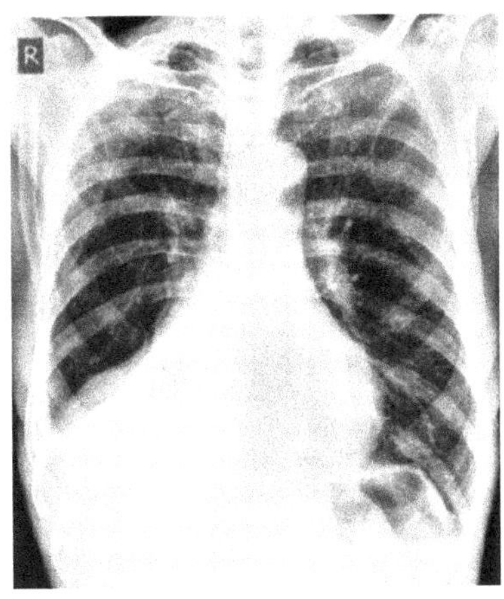

CHEST X-RAY 37

- *Description*: Left whole lung homogeneous opacity with trachea shifted to left side with elevation of left hemidiaphragm and heart border could not be delineated.
- *Differential diagnosis*:
    - Left sided whole lung collapse
    - Pulmonary agenesis
    - Left pneumonectomy
    - Rarely pleural mesothelioma (uncommon)
- *Final impression*: Left whole lung collapse

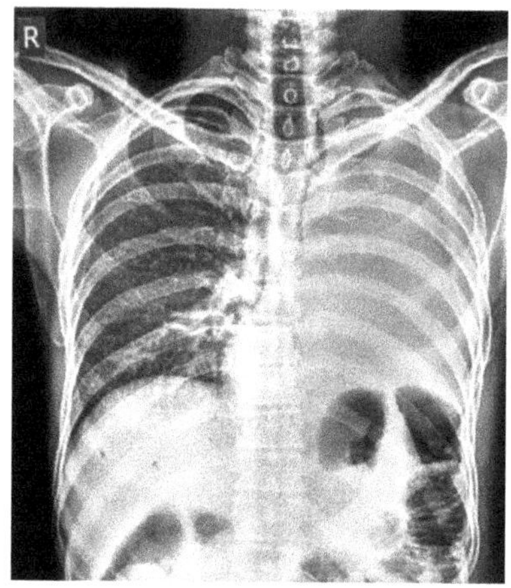

CHEST X-RAY 38

- *Description*: Right upper zone homogeneous opacity with erosion of part of right 1st and 2nd rib.
- *Differential diagnosis*:
    - Right sided pancoast tumor
    - Pulmonary TB with TB osteomyelitis of right 1st and 2nd rib
    - Secondary deposit in right apical region with rib erosion
- *Final impression*: Right sided pancoast tumor with erosion of 1st and 2nd rib.

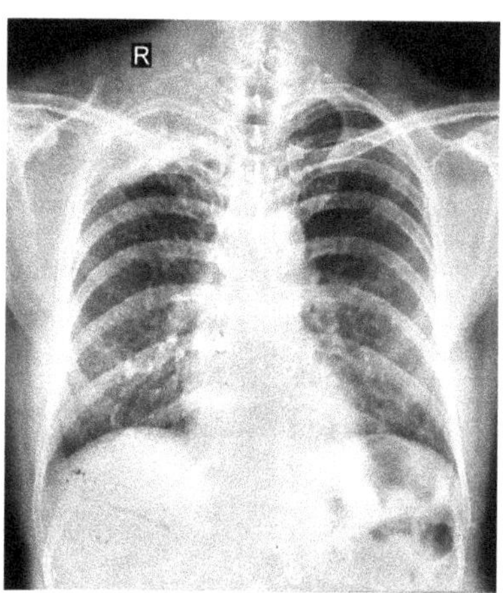

CHEST X-RAY 39

- *Right upper lobe collapse*: golden S sign
- Medial part bulge due to mass and lateral part elevated due to collapse of right upper lobe with elevation of transverse fissure.

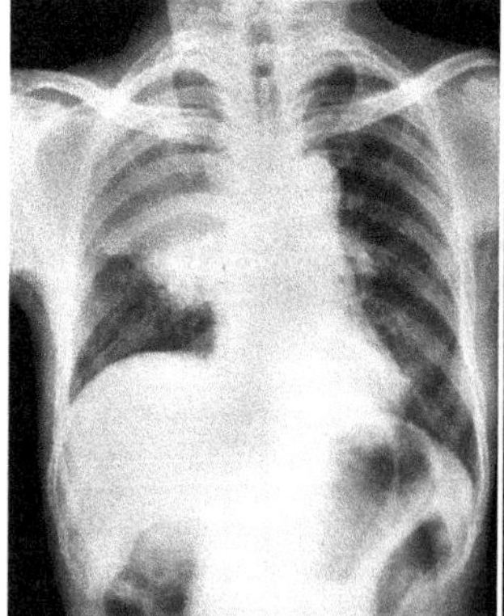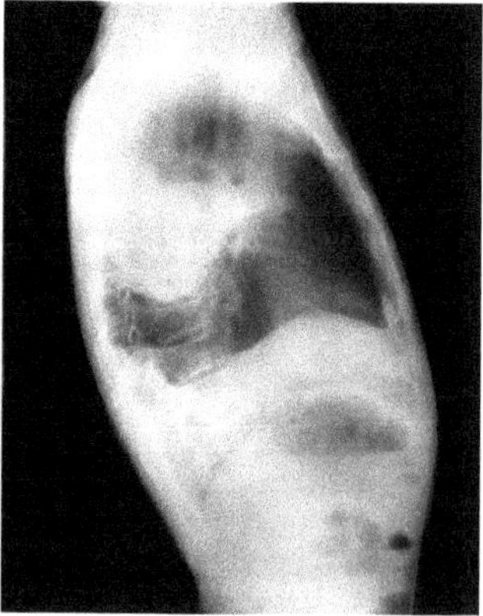

CHEST X-RAY 40

- *Description*: Right parahilar opacity with right lower zone thick walled irregular cavity.
- *Differential diagnosis*:
  - Endobronchial mass with hilar lymphadenopathy with distal pneumonia with breakdown
  - Right lower zone pyogenic cavity
  - Right lower zone tubercular cavity with right hilar lymphadenopathy
- *Final impression*: Endobronchial mass with hilar lymphadenopathy with distal pneumonia with breakdown.

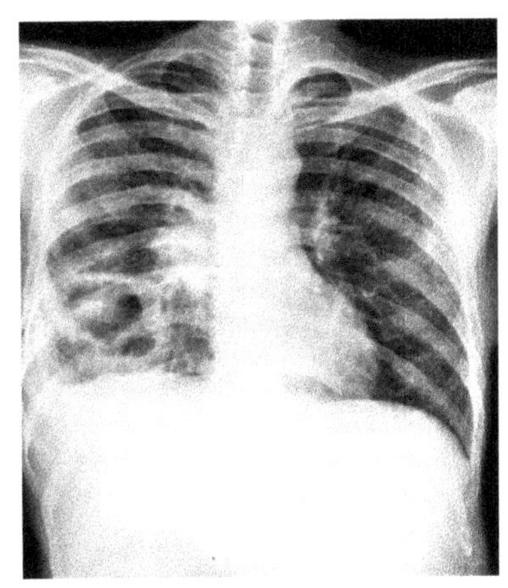

CHEST X-RAY 41

- *Description*: Lung abscess in right upper and mid zone with thick and irregular upper border of abscess cavity with elevation of right hemidiaphragm.
- *Differential diagnosis*:
  - Malignant cavity with phrenic nerve palsy
  - Bacterial lung abscess
  - Fungal lung abscess
  - Tubercular lung abscess
- *Final impression*: Malignant cavity with right phrenic nerve palsy.

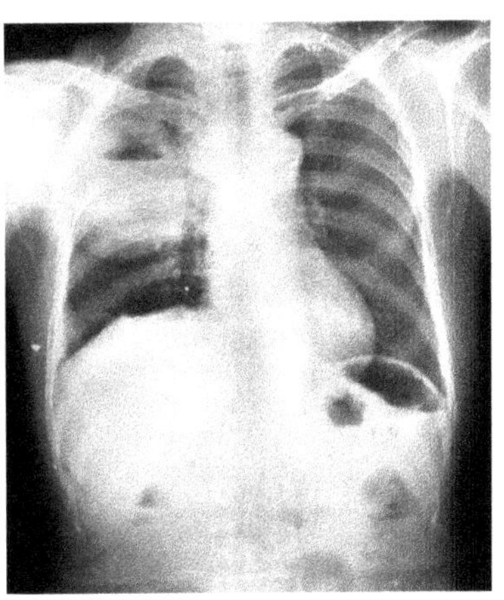

CHEST X-RAY 42

- Homogeneous opacity in left mid and lower zone with small air fluid level.
- *Differential diagnosis*:
  - Lung abscess
  - Subdiaphragmatic abscess
  - Eventration of diaphragm
  - Malignant lung abscess
- *Final impression*: Malignant lung abscess

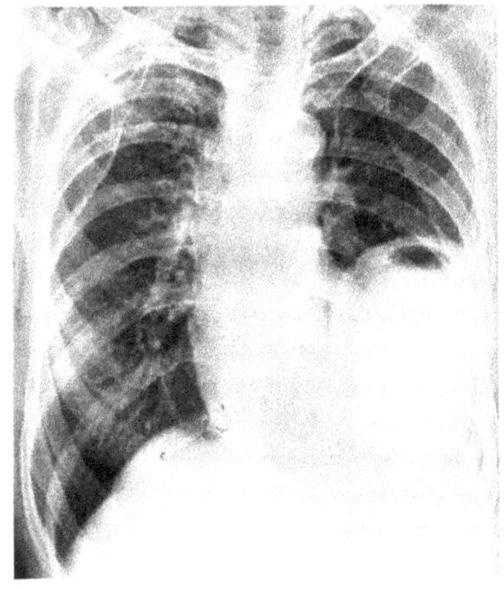

CHEST X-RAY 43

- *Description*: Superior mediastinal widening
- *Differential diagnosis*: Mediastinal lymphadeno-pathy

  Due to:
  - Lymphoma
  - TB
  - Secondary deposits in mediastinal lymph node
- Mediastinal widening: >6 cm in upright PA view, >8 cm in anteroposterior (AP) supine at the level of t4.
- *Final impression*: Lymphoma

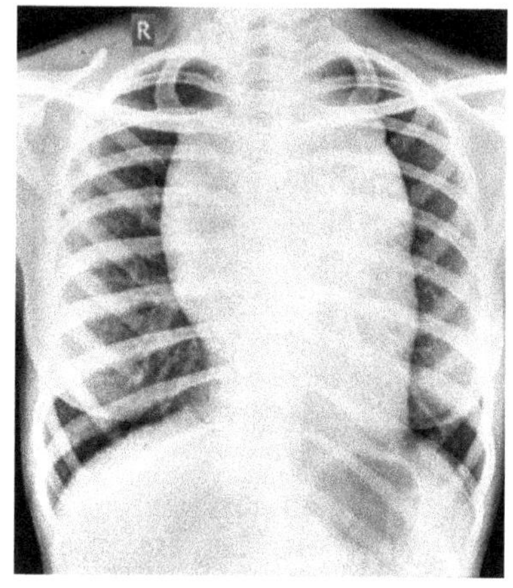

CHEST X-RAY 44

- *Description*: Entire right hemithorax homogeneous opacity with mediastinal shifting to opposite side.
- *Differential diagnosis*:
  - Right sided massive pleural effusion with mediastinal shifting to the opposite side
  - Right sided huge lung mass
  - Right sided large mediastinal mass with pleural effusion
- *Final impression*: Large mediastinal mass with right sided pleural effusion.

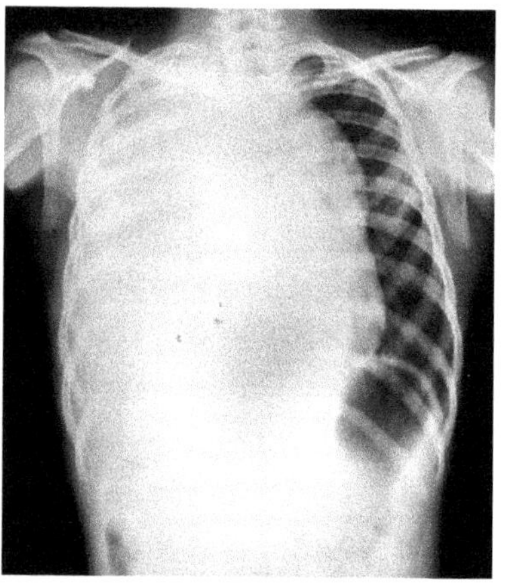

CHEST X-RAY 45

- *Description*: Left paratracheal, parahilar, paracardiac homogeneous opacity with undulation indicates mediastinal lymphadenopathy.
- *Differential diagnosis*:
  - Lymphoma
  - Lymph node metastasis
  - TB
  - Fungal disease
  - Sarcoidosis
- *Final impression*: Lymphoma

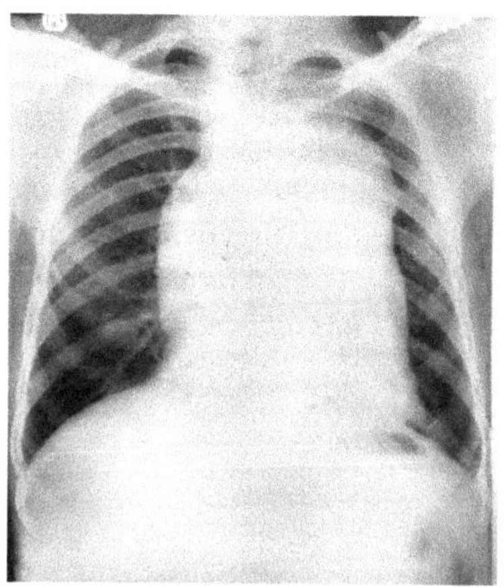

CHEST X-RAY 46

- *Description*:
  - Left upper zone air fluid level
  - Increased translucency in left lower zone with absence of bronchovascular markings
  - Outline of left hemidiaphragm is obscured
- *Differential diagnosis*:
  - Left sided multiple encysted hydropneumothorax
  - Left sided diaphragmatic hernia
- *Final impression*: Left sided diaphragmatic hernia

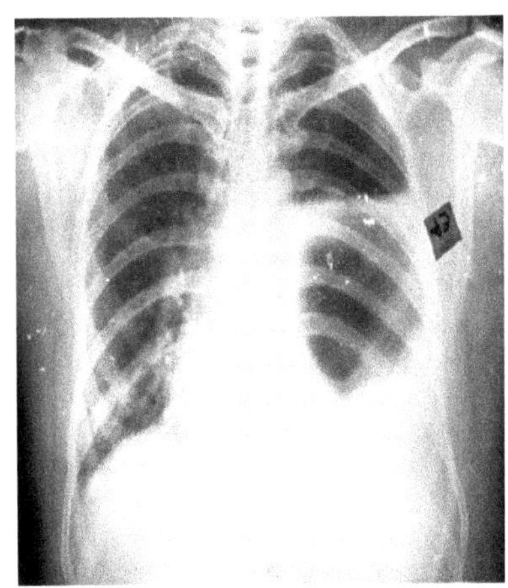

CHEST X-RAY 47

- *Description*: Opacity with air fluid level in right paracardiac area.
- *Differential diagnosis*:
  - Right sided lung abscess
  - Morgagni hernia
- *Final impression*: Morgagni hernia

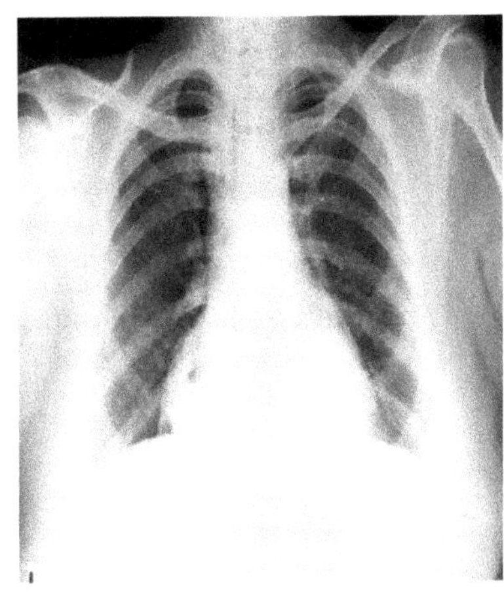

CHEST X-RAY 48

- *Description*: Presence of intestine in both lower zone but mainly on right lower zone.
- *Impression*:
  - A large defect in anterior aspect of median and paramedian location. Herniation of antrum, pylorus, multiple small bowel loops, hepatic flexure, and ascending and transverse colon with mesentery and omentum.
  - Mass effect in form of partial collapse of right middle lobe and right lower lobe with shift of heart to left.
  - Confirmed by contrast-enhanced computed tomography (CECT) thorax + CECT whole abdomen (oral + contrast).

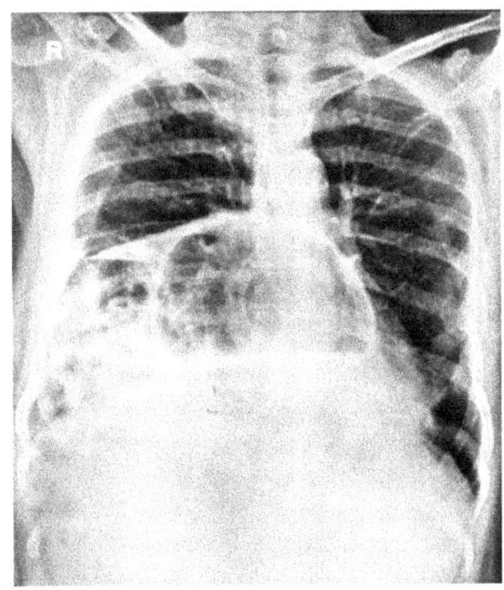

CHEST X-RAY 49

- *Description*: Air fluid level in left lower zone with shifting of heart to the right side.
- *Differential diagnosis*:
  - Left sided lung abscess
  - Left sided encysted hydropneumothorax
  - Eventration/hernia of left hemidiaphragm
  - Left sided subphrenic abscess
- *Final impression*: Eventration of left hemidiaphragm

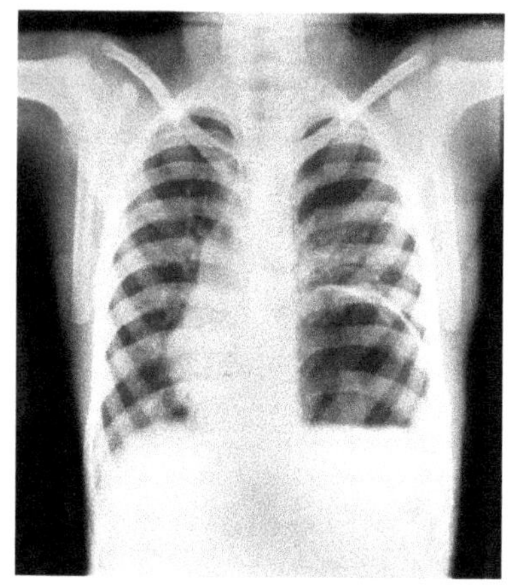

CHEST X-RAY 50

- *Description*: Homogeneous opacity with air fluid level seen in right lower zone with obliteration of right diaphragmatic margin.
- *Differential diagnosis*:
  - Lung abscess right lower zone
  - Subdiaphragmatic abscess—right
  - Liver abscess
- *Final impression*: Subdiaphragmatic abscess

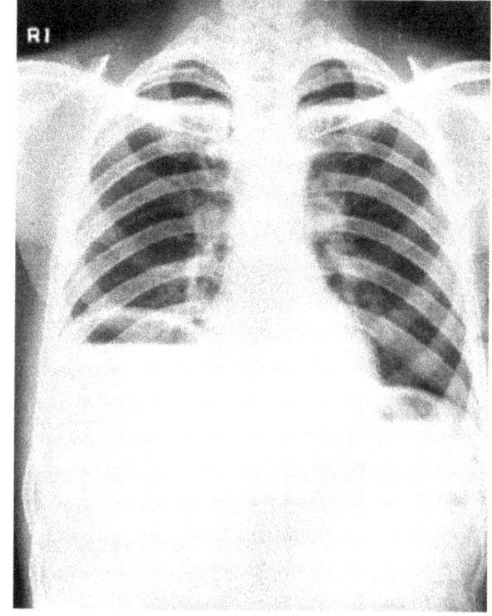

CHEST X-RAY 51

- *Description*: Heart shadow in the right side with fundal gas shadow in the right side.
- *Final impression*: Dextrocardia with situs inversus.

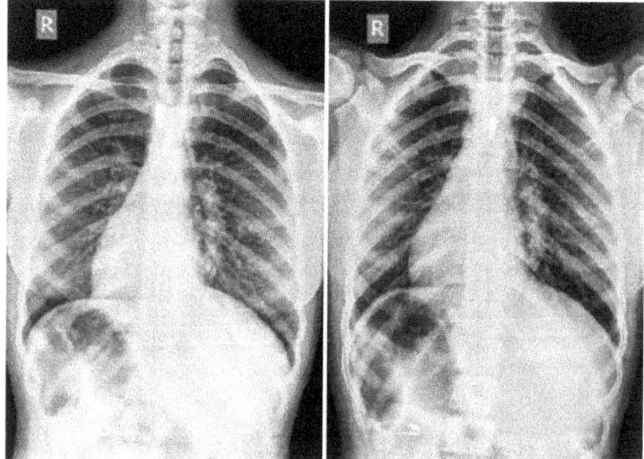

CHEST X-RAY 52

- *Description*: Increased cardiac silhouette
- *Differential diagnosis*:
  - Pericardial effusion
  - Dilated cardiomyopathy
  - Multivalvular heart disease with heart failure
  - Hypertensive heart failure
- *Final impression*: Pericardial effusion

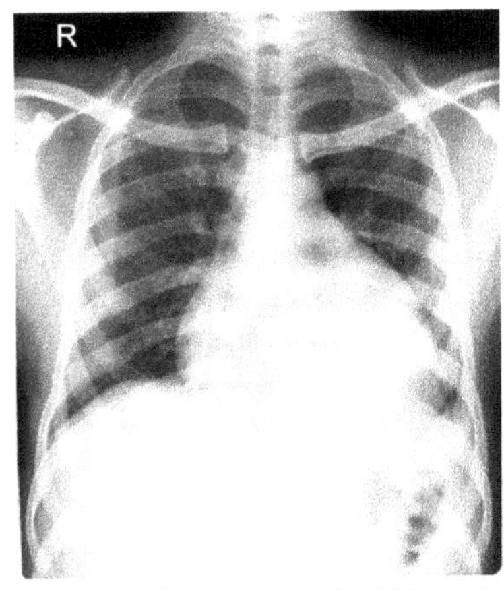

CHEST X-RAY 53

- *Description*: Calcified pericardium
- *Final impression*: TB of pericardium with sequelae

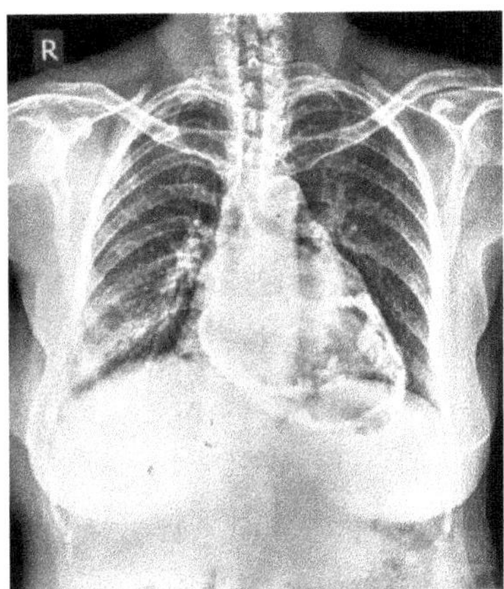

CHEST X-RAY 54

- *Description*: Bilateral extensive paracardiac, paratracheal nonhomogeneous opacity (r > l) with fullness of pulmonary bay.
- *Final impression*: Congenital heart disease with bilateral pulmonary plethora (r > l) with pulmonary arterial hypertension.

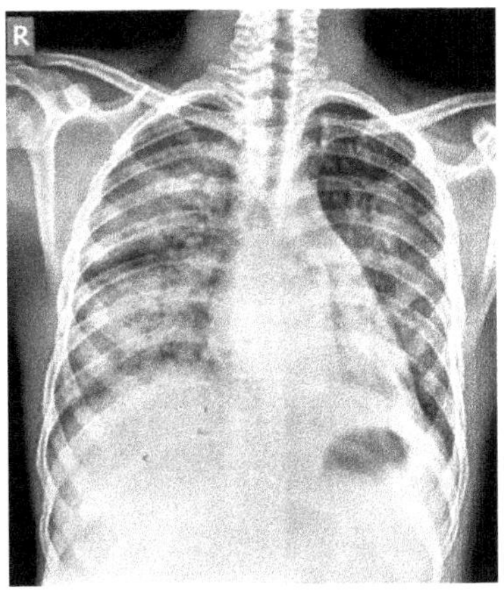

CHEST X-RAY 55

- *Description*: Right sided paratracheal shadow with increased cardiothoracic (c-t) ratio
- *Differential diagnosis*: Right sided aortic arch with boot shaped heart [right ventricular hypertrophy (RVH)]
- *Final Impression*: Right sided aortic arch with right ventricular hypertrophy (echo proved Fallot's tetralogy)

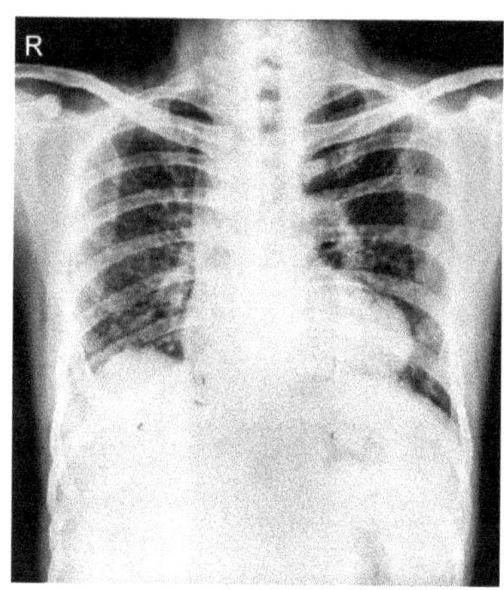

CHEST X-RAY 56

- *Description*: Left paratracheal shadow with well-defined margin.
- *Differential diagnosis*:
    - Aneurysm of arch of aorta
    - Mediastinal mass
    - Mediastinal lymphadenopathy
- *Final impression*: Aneurysm of arch of aorta

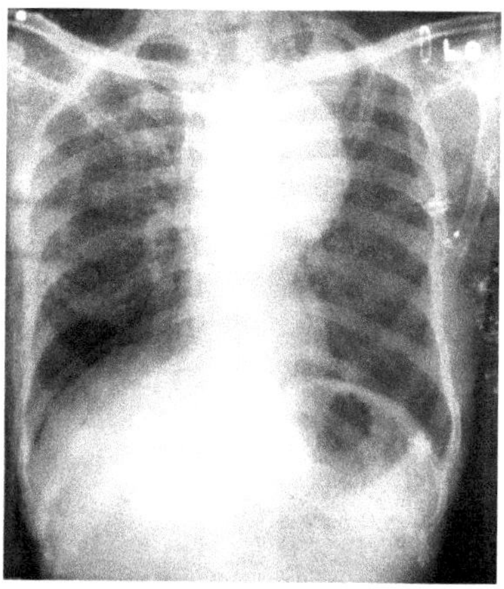

CHEST X-RAY 57

- *Description*: Homogeneous opacity in right lower zone and homogeneous opacity in right mid zone with water lily sign.
- *Final impression*: Ruptured hydatid cyst in right mid zone and another unruptured hydatid cyst in right lower zone.

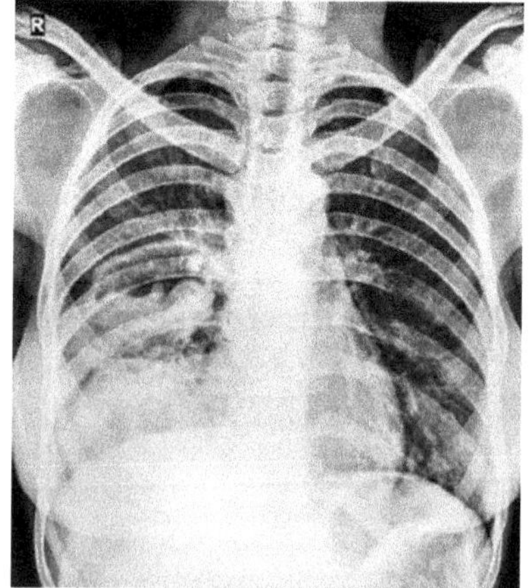

CHEST X-RAY 58

- *Description*: Normal bronchography of right lung.
- *Indications of bronchography*: Previously, it was the gold standard investigation for diagnosis of bronchiectasis.

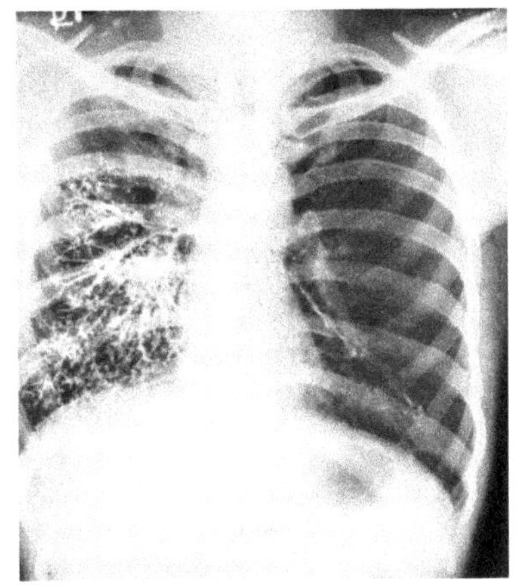

CHEST X-RAY 59

- *Description*: Left sided, mid and lower part of rib cage medially displaced with left sided lower part volume loss.
- *Impression*: A case of left sided thoracoplasty with left upper lobe predominant scattered parenchymal fibrosis.
- *Thoracoplasty*: Removing or resecting one or more ribs to obliterate the lung cavity and collapse of the diseased part.

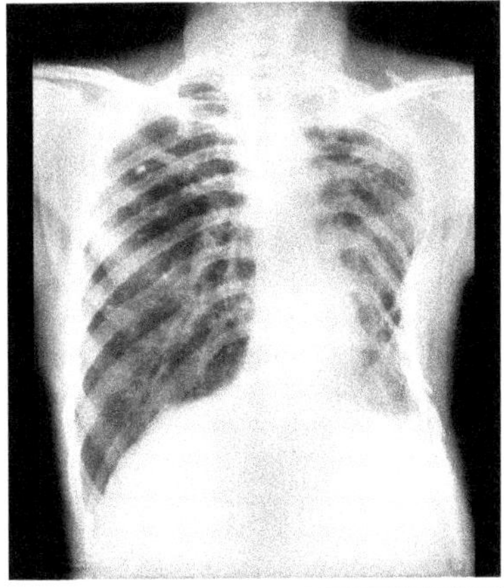

CHEST X-RAY 60

- Few ribs are cut to obliterate left upper lobe cavity for treatment of recurrent massive hemoptysis—thoracoplasty.
- *Final impression*: Thoracoplasty of upper part of left lung.

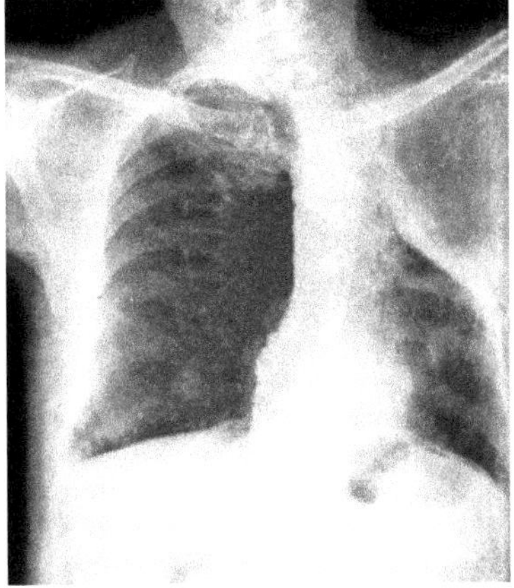

CHEST X-RAY 61

- *Description*: Barium swallow esophagus with significant narrowing with irregular margin in lower part and dilated upper part.
- *Final impression*: Esophageal carcinoma

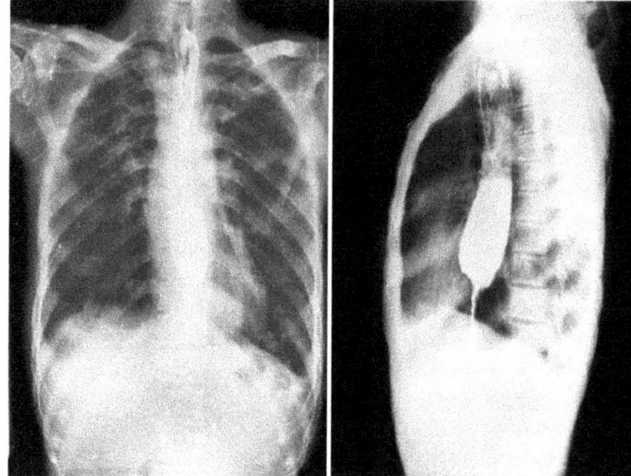

CHEST X-RAY 62

- *Description*: Multiple nodular shadows over the ribs.
- *Differential diagnosis*: Bilateral multiple rib fracture with callous formation (of some duration).

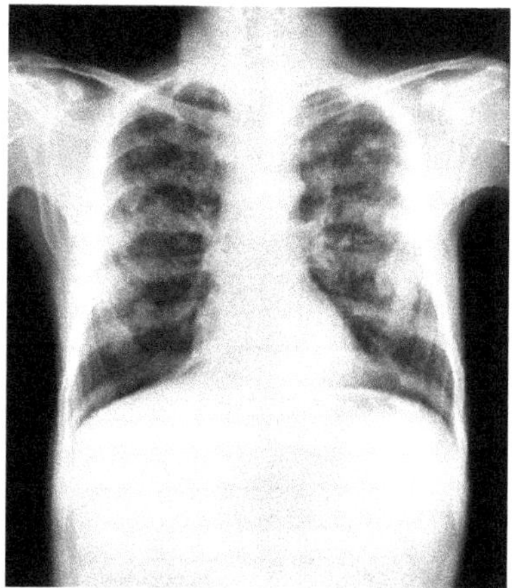

CHEST X-RAY 63

- *Intestinal coil under right diaphragm*: Chilaiditi syndrome
- This syndrome is a benign condition in which a segment of the intestine is interposed between liver and diaphragm.

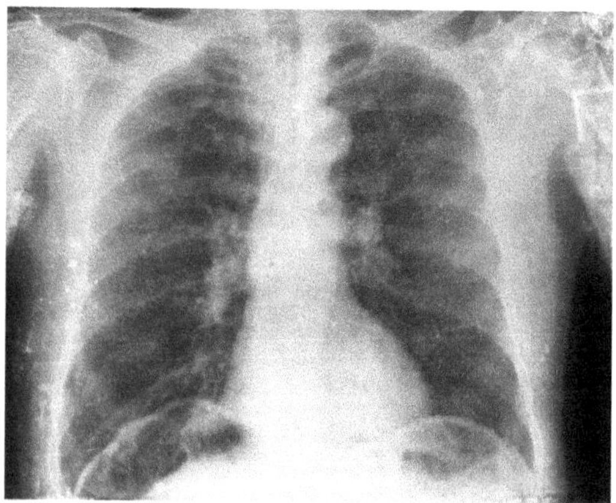

EXERCISES

EXERCISE 1

- *Description*: Right mid zone homogeneous round opacity
- *Differential diagnosis*:
  - Hydatid cyst
  - Bronchial cyst
  - Lung abscess before rupture
  - Benign lung mass
  - Encysted pleural effusion
- *Final impression*: Hydatid cyst

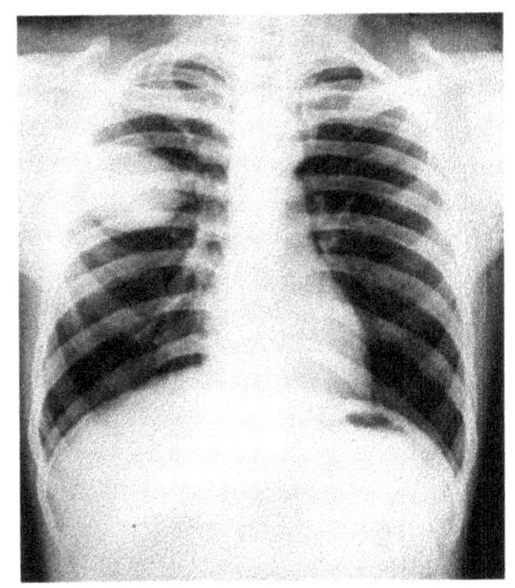

EXERCISE 2

- *Description*: Right upper lobe homogeneous opacity with bulging of medial end of transverse fissure and upward displacement of transverse fissure in the lateral part.
- *Impression*: Right upper lobe mass with right upper lobe collapse—medial bulging is due to mass and upward displacement of transverse fissure in the lateral part is due to collapse (golden S sign).

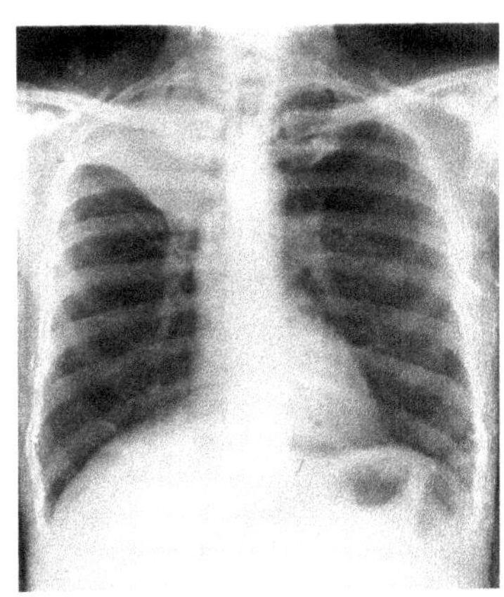

EXERCISE 3

- *Description*: Homogeneous opacity in right upper zone with destruction of right 1st rib.
- *Differential diagnosis*:
  - Pancoast tumor
  - Right upper zone pulmonary TB with osteomyelitis of right 1st rib
- *Final impression*: Superior sulcus tumor.

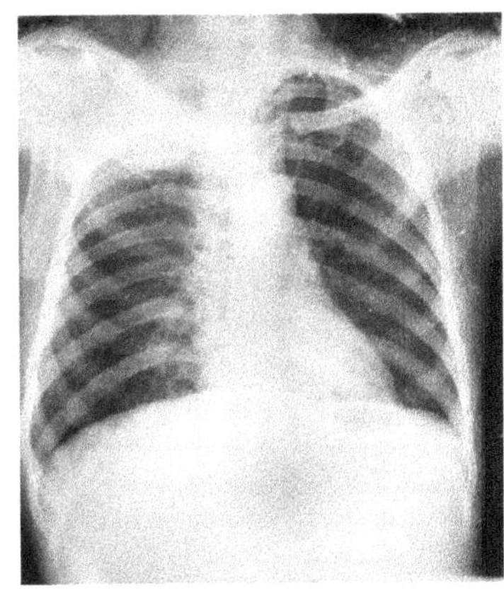

EXERCISE 4

- *Description*: Increased cardiac silhouette
- *Differential diagnosis*:
  - Pericardial effusion
  - Dilated cardiomyopathy
- *Final impression*: Mild pericardial effusion

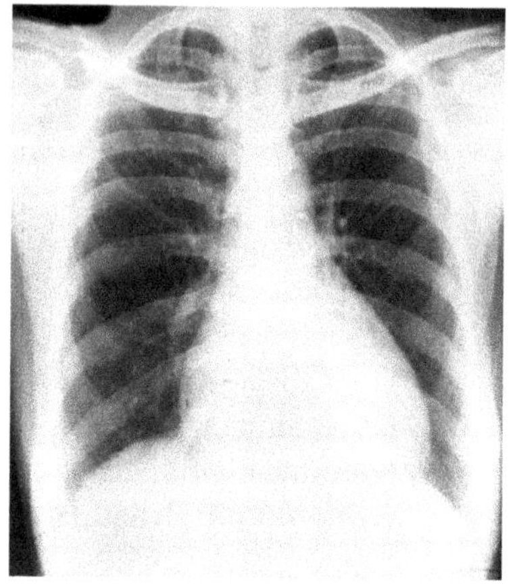

EXERCISE 5

- *Description*: Dilatation of aortic arch
- *Differential diagnosis*:
  - Left sided mediastinal mass
  - Left lung mass
  - Aneurysm of aortic arch
- *Final impression*: Aneurysm of aortic arch

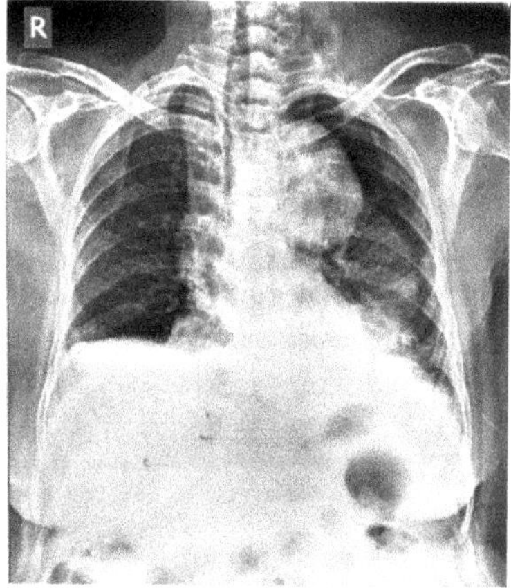

EXERCISE 6

- Bilateral lower zone cavities with left water lily sign and right handkerchief sign
- *Final impression*: Bilateral ruptured hydatid cyst.

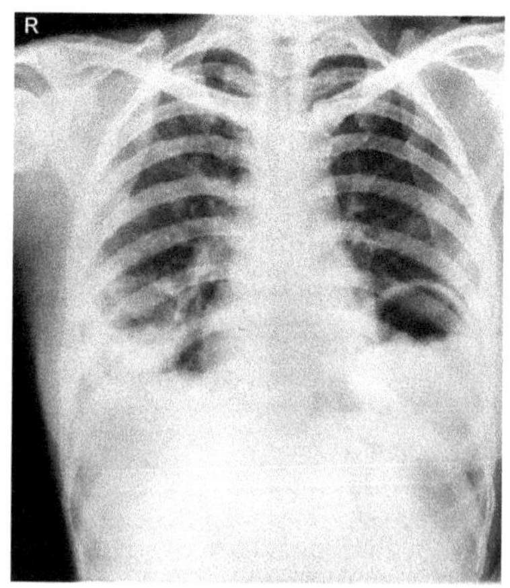

EXERCISE 7

- Left sided thoracoplasty

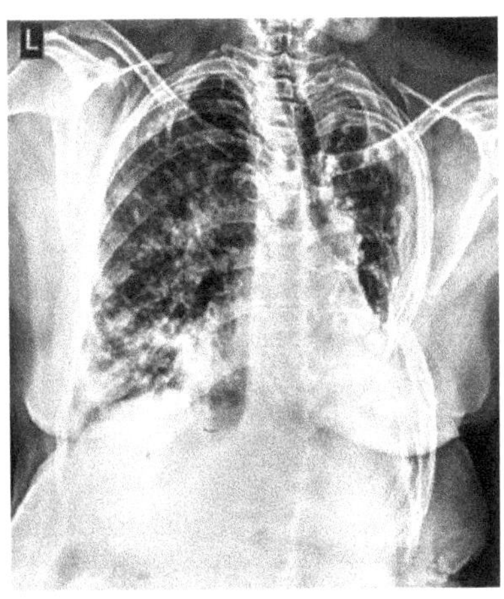

EXERCISE 8

- *Description*: Bilateral multiple parenchymal calcification varying in shape and predominantly on the right side with right sided pleural thickening.
- *Differential diagnosis*: Healed calcified foci with right sided pleural thickening—post TB sequelae.

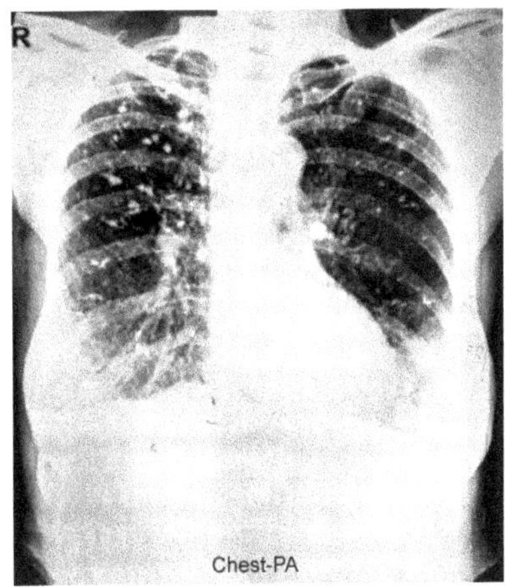

Computed Tomography Scan of Thorax

Susmita Kundu

BASIC PRINCIPLES OF COMPUTED TOMOGRAPHY SCAN

- Computed tomography (CT) is based on the fundamental principle that the density of the tissue passed by the X-ray beam can be measured from the calculation of the attenuation coefficient. Using this principle, CT allows the reconstruction of the density of the body, by two-dimensional section perpendicular to the axis of the acquisition system.
- Hounsfield chose a scale that affects the four basic densities, with the following values:
  1. Air = –1,000
  2. Fat = –60 to –120
  3. Water = 0
  4. Compact bone = +1,000

INDICATIONS OF COMPUTED TOMOGRAPHY THORAX

- To confirm the abnormalities found on conventional chest X-ray (CXR).
- To evaluate the clinical signs or symptoms of diseases of the chest, such as cough, shortness of breath, and hemoptysis.
- To evaluate diffuse parenchymal lung disease (DPLD).
- To assess improvement or deterioration of pulmonary diseases following treatment.
- To detect and evaluate lung tumors.
- To assess whether the tumors are responding to treatment or not.
- To evaluate injury to chest.

HIGH-RESOLUTION COMPUTED TOMOGRAPHY TECHNIQUE

- *Slice thickness:* ≤2 mm for nonhelical CT ≤1.5 mm for helical CT.
- High spatial frequency reconstruction algorithm.
- Scan time as short as possible (0.3–0.5 seconds).
- Axial or helical mode of data acquisition.
- Kilovoltage peak (kVp) and milli-Ampere (mA) both per slice as well as optimized for volumetric data acquisition.
- Patient positioning (supine and/or prone).
- State of respiration (inspiration and/or expiration).

SALIENT ANATOMY (FIG. 1)

- Secondary pulmonary lobule is a polyhedral structure (around 2 cm diameter) with bronchovascular structures in the center and perilobular veins (peripheral interstitium) in the periphery.
- Lymphatics are seen in the center as well as periphery of the lobule.
- Each secondary pulmonary lobule is supplied by a terminal bronchiole and a centrilobular pulmonary artery.
- Terminal bronchiole is thin, does not have any cilia but has muscular wall which makes them a favored location for bronchospasm leading to air trapping.
- Terminal bronchioles give rise to multiple respiratory bronchioles which lead to alveolar ducts.
- Bronchovascular bundle consists of bronchi/bronchioles, arteries, and associated connective tissue.

PATTERNS AND TERMINOLOGIES

Reticular Pattern

- This is one of the commonly seen abnormalities in interstitial lung disease (ILD).
- It manifests as linear opacities on high-resolution computed tomography (HRCT) as a result of thickening of the peripheral interstitium especially interlobular septum.
- Reticular pattern can be smooth, nodular, and irregular.
- Nodular reticular opacities are seen in sarcoidosis, pneumoconiosis, lymphangitis carcinomatosis, and hypersensitivity pneumonitis (HP).
- Irregular reticular pattern as a result of extensive interstitial fibrosis leading to irregular thickening of septae and pulmonary lobule. This pattern is seen in fibrosing ILD such as fibrotic nonspecific interstitial pneumonia (NSIP), usual interstitial pneumonia (UIP), and sarcoidosis.

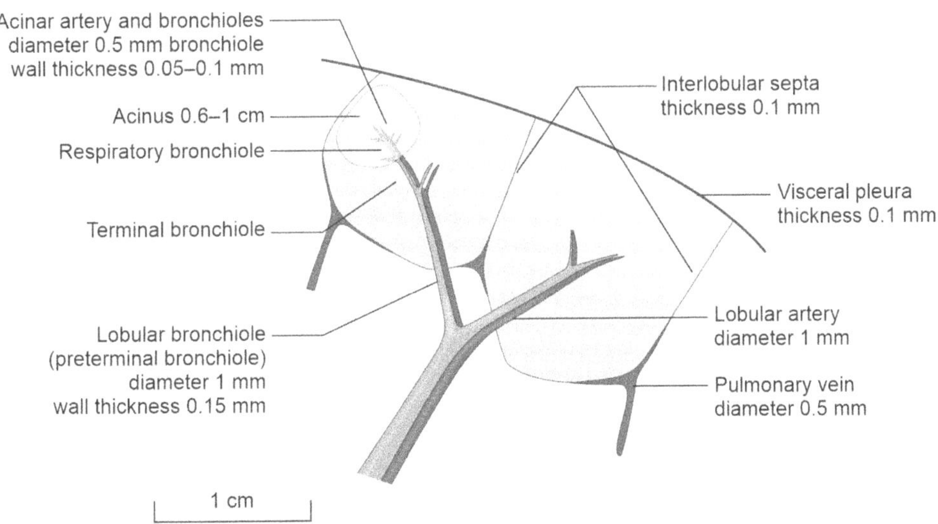

FIG. 1: Anatomy of secondary pulmonary lobule.

Nodular Pattern

- This pattern consists of discrete nodules of varying size—micronodular (<3 mm), macronodular (3–10 mm) distributed in the pulmonary lobule, single nodule up to 30 mm is solitary pulmonary nodule (SPN).
- Causes may be granulomatous disease, pneumoconiosis, metastasis, etc.
- Centrilobular, perilymphatic, and random—these three types of nodules are distributed in the secondary lobule.
- Perilymphatic nodules are seen along the peripheral interstitium which means nodules are seen along the pleura and fissures on HRCT, e.g., sarcoidosis and other granulomatous diseases.
- Random nodules will not follow any particular pattern of distribution in secondary pulmonary lobule, e.g., miliary tuberculosis (TB), metastasis, etc.

Ground Glass Opacity and Consolidation Pattern

- Consolidation is an abnormal increase in lung density with effacement of pulmonary vessels while in ground glass opacity (GGO) there is no effacement of pulmonary vessels and consolidation also leads to opacification of pulmonary spaces and/or interstitium.
- Alveolar pattern can be seen in acute interstitial pneumonia, acute respiratory distress syndrome (ARDS), *Pneumocystis jirovecii* pneumonia (PJP), bronchoalveolar carcinoma (CA), alveolar hemorrhage, etc.
- Mosaic attenuation is commonly associated with patchy areas of increased/decreased lucency leading to heterogeneous appearance of lung parenchyma due to abnormalities in small airway, peripheral pulmonary vasculature or interstitium.
- Tree in bud pattern is a manifestation of endobronchial spread of infection such as TB or aspiration and characterized by linear branching structures (opacified distal bronchioles) with nodular opacities (acinar).

Cystic Pattern

- Cystic lesions in lung are usually formed by the abnormal dilatation of bronchi/bronchioles.
- Patterns of cystic lesion may look such as cluster of grapes, string of pearls, honey combing, and random cysts.
- Clusters of grapes seen in cystic bronchiectasis due to abnormal dilatation of airways involving a lobe or segment.
- Air fluid level in cystic lesion indicates secondary infection.
- String of pearl pattern is characterized by the presence of multiple cysts in a single row along the pleura.
- Honey combing is relatively smaller thick-walled cysts arranged in multiple layers, seen in fibrosing ILDs.
- Centriacinar emphysema, pulmonary Langerhans cell histiocytosis (PLCH), and leiomyomatosis may present with randomly distributed cysts.

COMPUTED TOMOGRAPHY THORAX 1

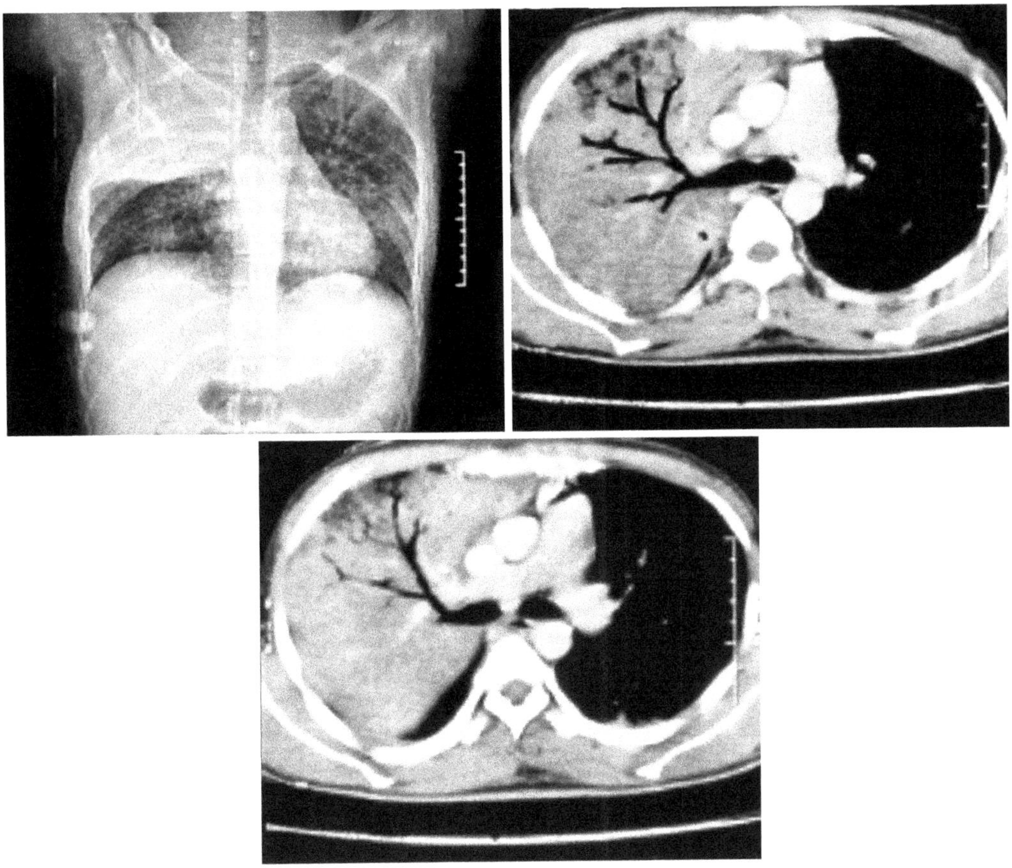

- *Description*: Right upper lobe pneumonia with air bronchogram with bulging fissure sign. Bulging fissure sign is classically seen in *Klebsiella pneumonia*.
- *Final impression*: Right upper lobe community acquired pneumonia.

COMPUTED TOMOGRAPHY THORAX 2A

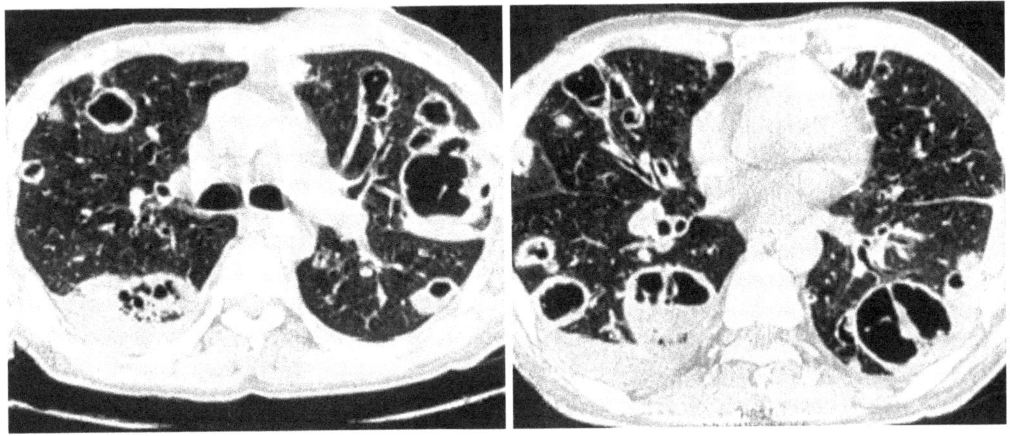

- *Description*: Bilateral infected cysts/bulla with right minimal pleural effusion and necrotizing pneumonia in right side.
- *Differential diagnosis*:
  - Pulmonary TB
  - Bacterial infection—staphylococcal
  - Cystic bronchiectasis
- *Final impression*: Multiple cavitary lesion following staphylococcal pneumonia.

CHEST X-RAY 2B

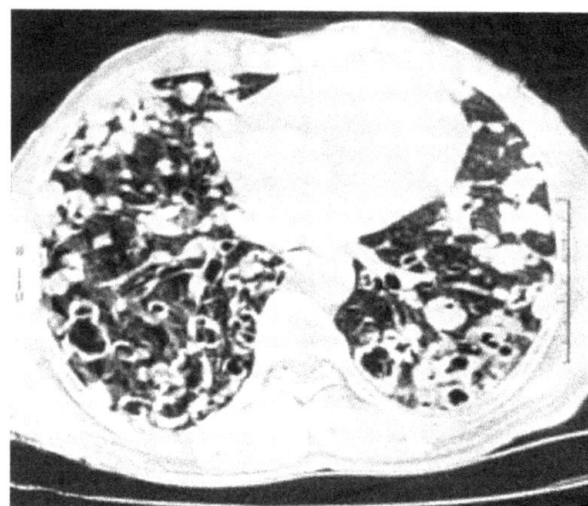
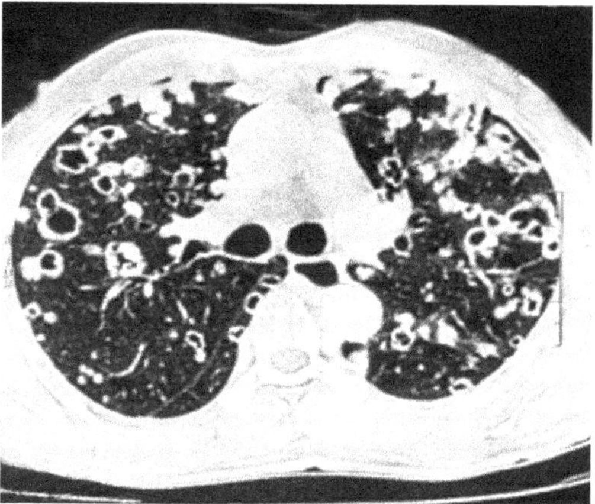

- *Description*: Bilateral extensive small cystic lesion involving all the lobes of lung and bilateral multiple micro and macro nodular opacities.
- *Differential diagnosis*:
  - Bacterial infection—staphylococcal
  - Fungal infection
  - Pulmonary TB
  - Pulmonary metastasis
- *Final impression*: Pneumatocele following to staph infection.

COMPUTED TOMOGRAPHY THORAX 3

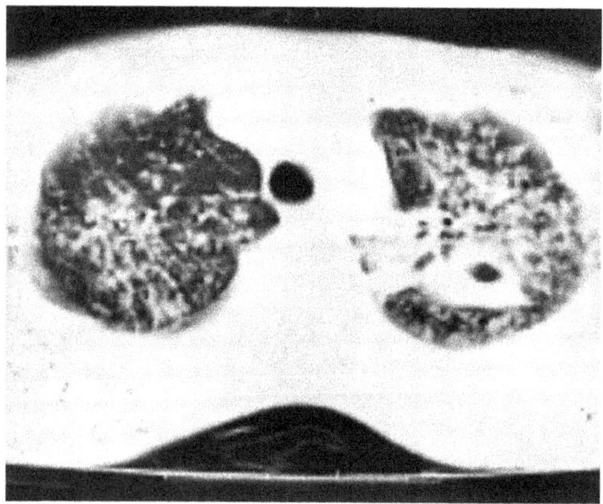
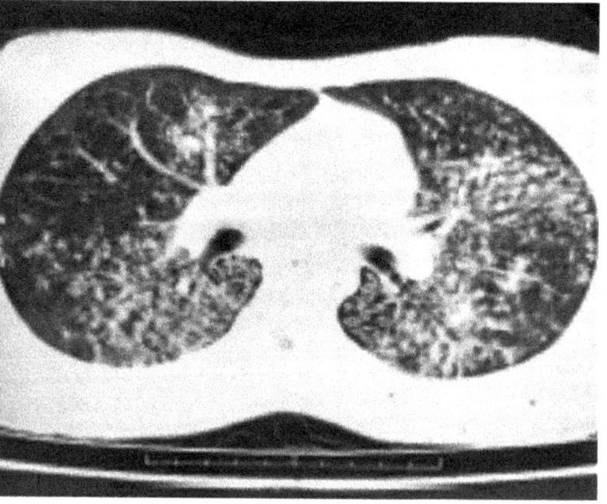

Continued

Continued

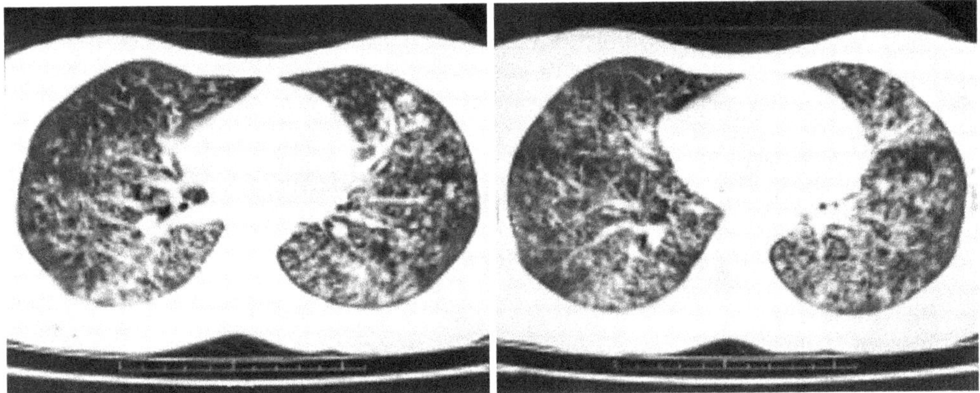

- *Description*: Bilateral extensive miliary shadow with tree in bud and cavity in left upper lobe.
- *Differential diagnosis*:
  - TB
  - Fungal infection
  - Silico-TB
  - Miliary metastasis
- *Final impression*: Pulmonary TB

COMPUTED TOMOGRAPHY THORAX 4

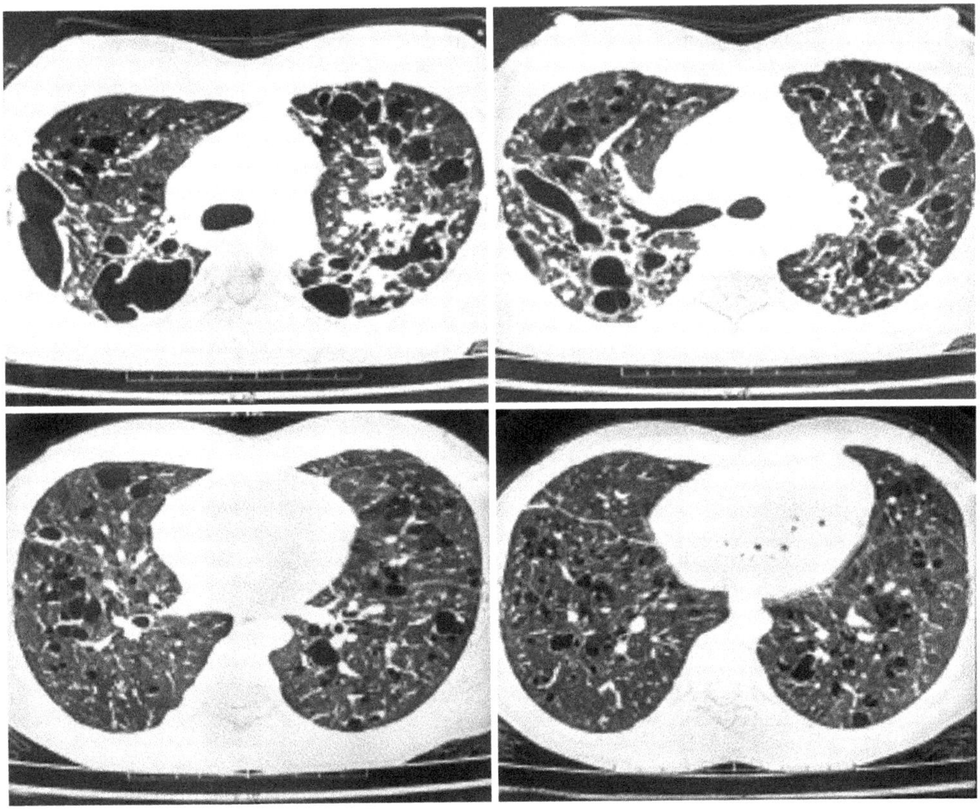

- *Description*: Bilateral extensive cystic lesion with bilateral upper lobe predominant fibrosis right > left (r>l) with paraseptal emphysema.
- *Differential diagnosis*:
  - PLCH
  - Lymphangioleiomyomatosis (LAM)
  - Post-TB sequelae
- *Final impression*: Pulmonary TB—proven by transbronchial lung biopsy (TBLB)

COMPUTED TOMOGRAPHY THORAX 5

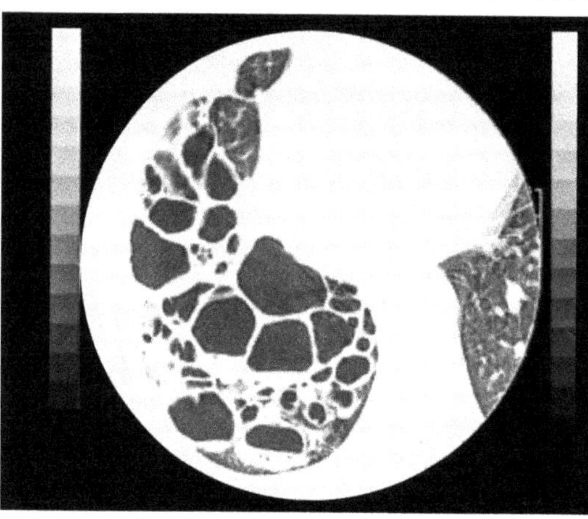
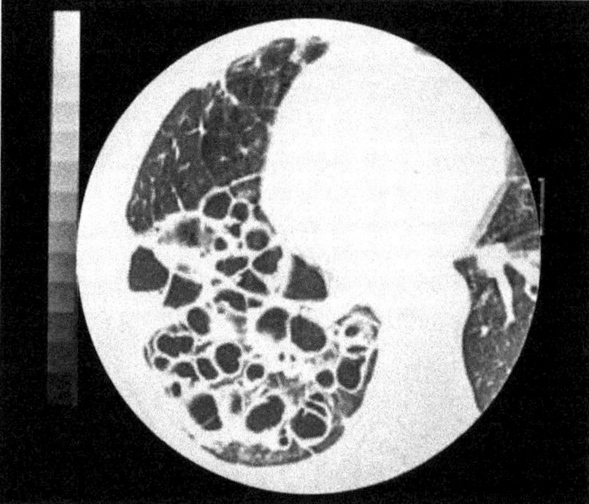

- *Description*: Right lower lobe cystic bronchiectasis.
- *Differential diagnosis*:
  - Following recurrent aspiration pneumonia
  - Post-tubercular sequelae
  - Following recurrent bacterial infection
- *Final impression*: Right lower lobe bronchiectasis due to recurrent bacterial infection since childhood.

COMPUTED TOMOGRAPHY THORAX 6

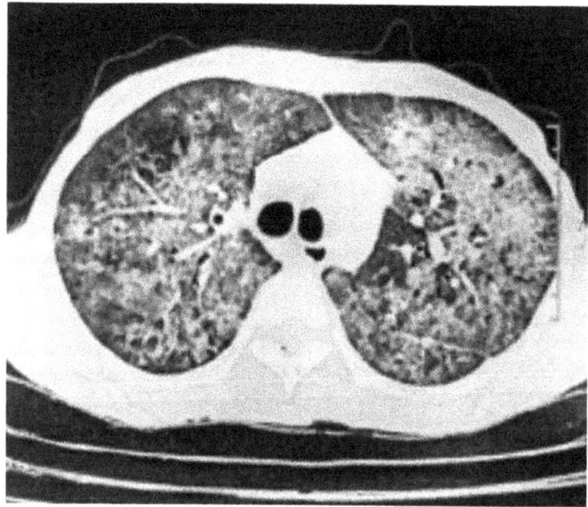
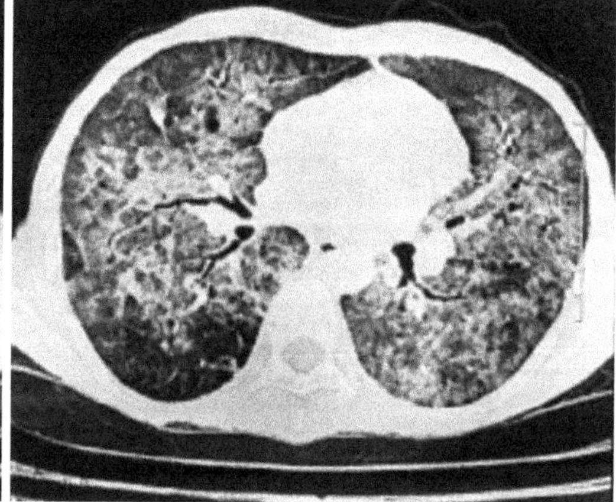

- *Description*: Bilateral paratracheal, parahilar, and paracardiac extensive GGO.
- *Differential diagnosis*:
  - ARDS
  - Heart failure
  - Acute interstitial pneumonia
  - Cryptogenic organizing pneumonia
  - Uremic lung
- *Final impression*: ARDS

COMPUTED TOMOGRAPHY THORAX 7

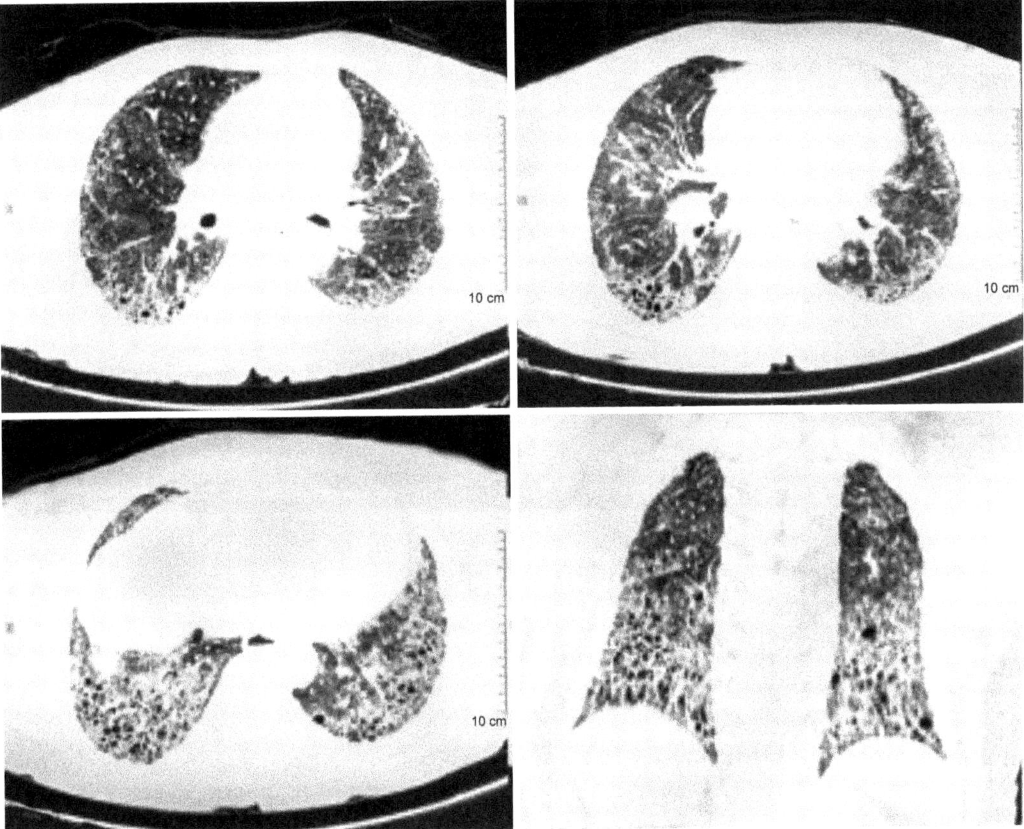

- *Description*: Bilateral, bibasal subpleural honey combing with traction bronchiectasis—UIP pattern. Straight edge sign—isolation of fibrosis to the lung bases with sharp demarcation in the craniocaudal plane without substantial extension along the lateral margins. It suggests collagen vascular disease.
- *Differential diagnosis*:
  - Connective tissue disease (CTD) related ILD
  - Occupational lung disease
  - Drug-induced ILD
  - Idiopathic pulmonary fibrosis (IPF)
- *Final impression*: CTD related ILD with UIP pattern.

COMPUTED TOMOGRAPHY THORAX 8

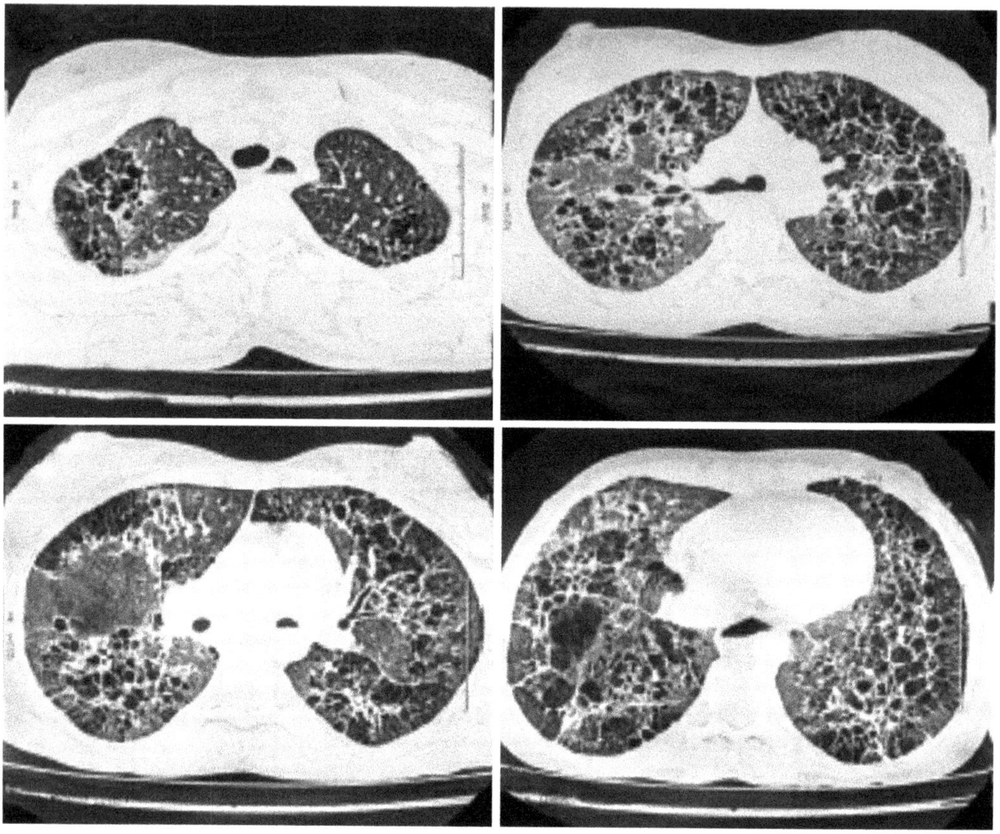

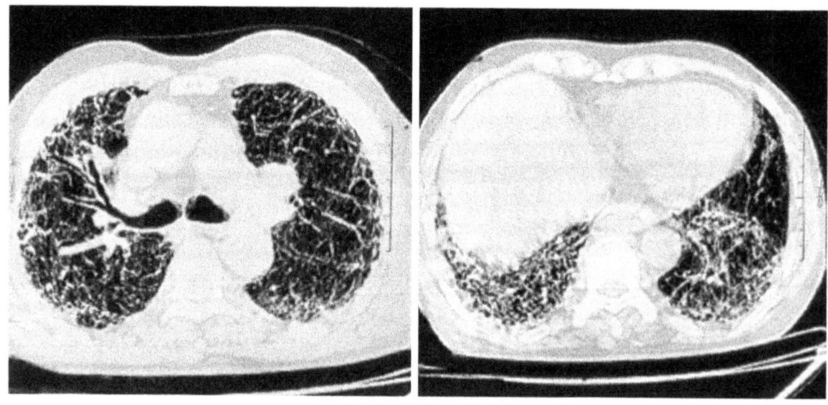

- *Description*: Bilateral extensive reticulation involving all the lobes with few cystic lesions (left) and traction bronchiectasis with GGO with bilateral subpleural honeycombing and dilated oesophagus.
- *Final impression*: Progressive system sclerosis—interstitial lung disease (PSS-ILD) (probable UIP pattern).

COMPUTED TOMOGRAPHY THORAX 9

- *Description*: Bilateral, bibasal subpleural honeycombing with reticulation and traction bronchiectasis—UIP pattern.
- *Final impression*: It is a case of IPF as no other cause detected.

▧ COMPUTED TOMOGRAPHY THORAX 10

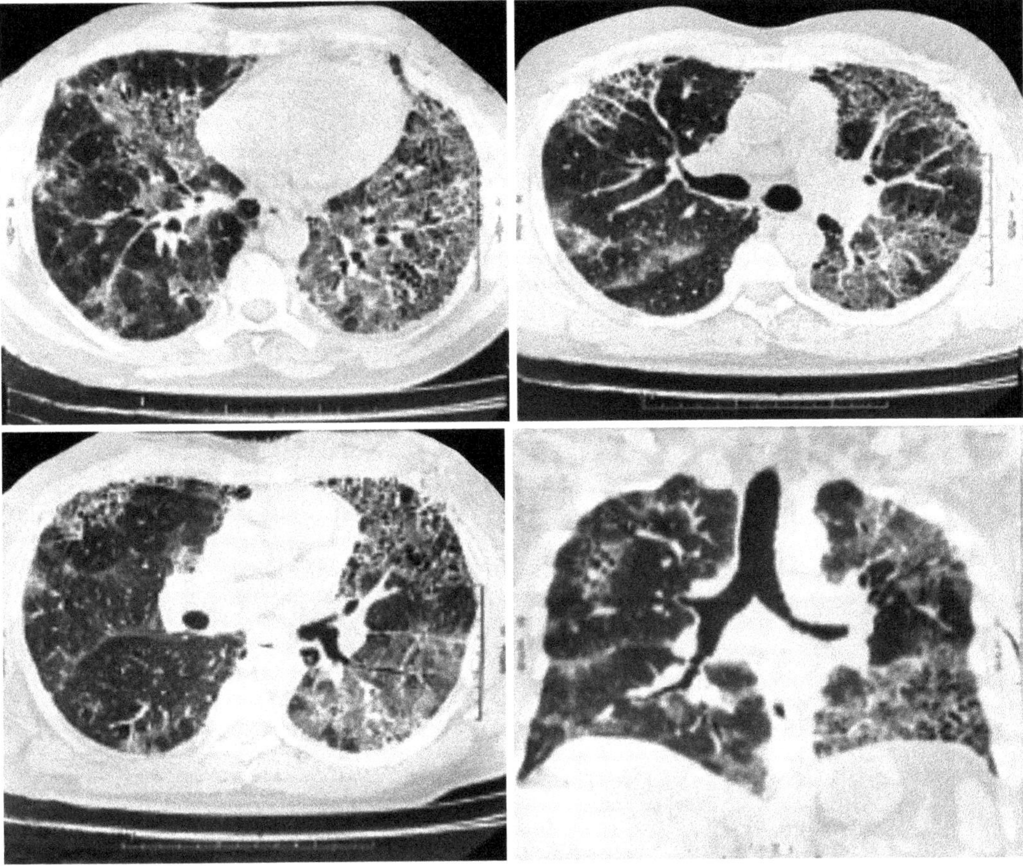

- *Description*: Bilateral extensive GGO with mosaic attenuation with reticulation and traction bronchiectasis—three density sign.
- *Three density sign*: Juxtaposition of lobular regions of low, normal, and high attenuation indicative of mixed infiltrative and obstructive process—suggestive of HP.
- *Final impression*: Chronic HP

COMPUTED TOMOGRAPHY THORAX 11

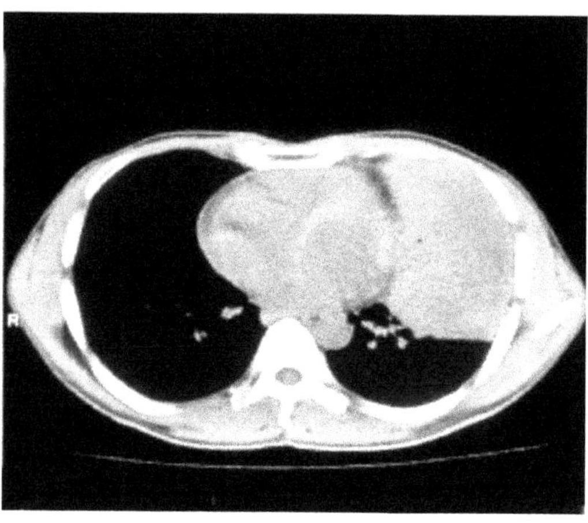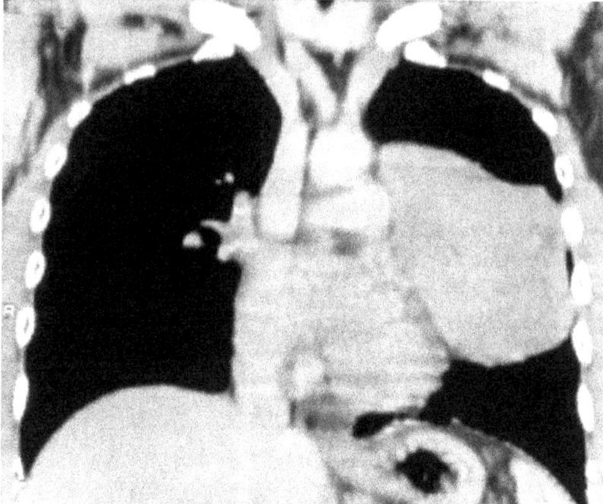

- *Description*: Homogeneous opacity occupying left lingular segment.
- *Differential diagnosis*:
    - Left lung malignancy
    - Left lung benign mass
    - Left upper lobe (lingular) pneumonia
- *Final impression*: Left lung mass in lingular segment.

COMPUTED TOMOGRAPHY THORAX 12A AND B

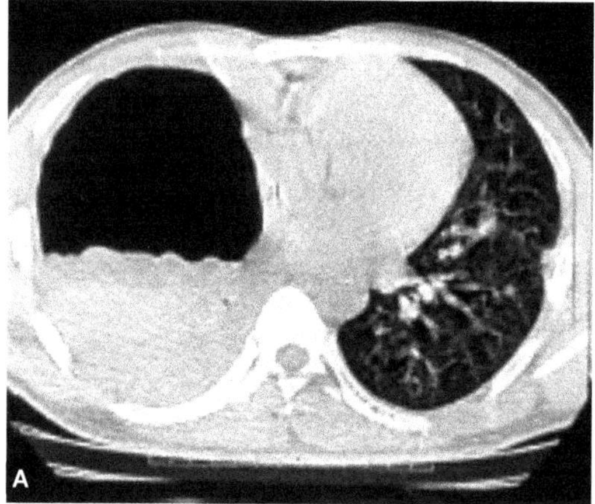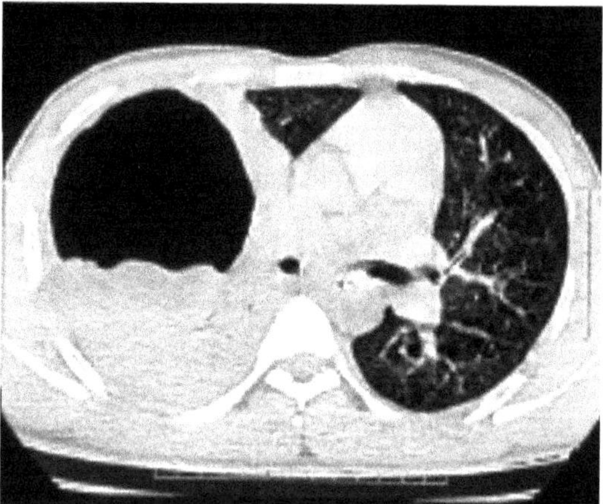

Continued

Continued

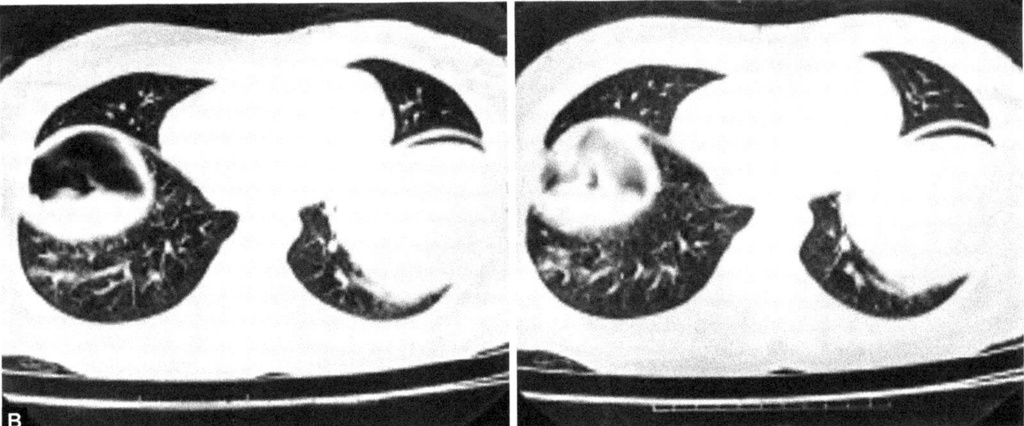

- *Description*: Right sided ruptured hydatid cyst—water lily (camolette) sign
- *Description*: Bilateral ruptured hydatid cyst water lily (camolette) sign on right side meniscus sign on left side.

COMPUTED TOMOGRAPHY THORAX 13

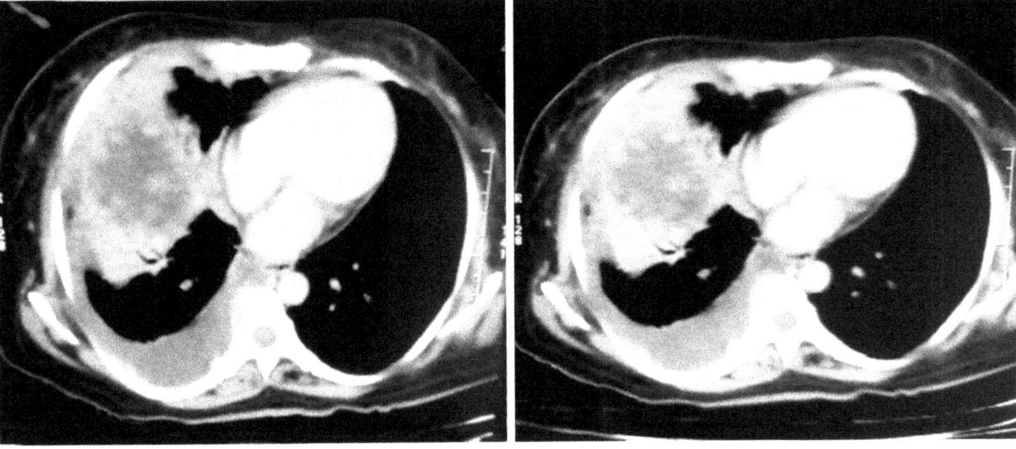

- *Description*: Right sided space occupying lesion (SOL) abutting the chest with central area of necrosis with multiple projections from the wall with right sided pleural effusion.
- *Differential diagnosis*:
    - Right sided malignant SOL
    - Right sided lung abscess
    - Right sided hydatid cyst with multiple daughter cysts
- *Final impression*: Right sided hydatid cyst with multiple daughter cysts—confirmed by echinococcal serology.

COMPUTED TOMOGRAPHY THORAX 14

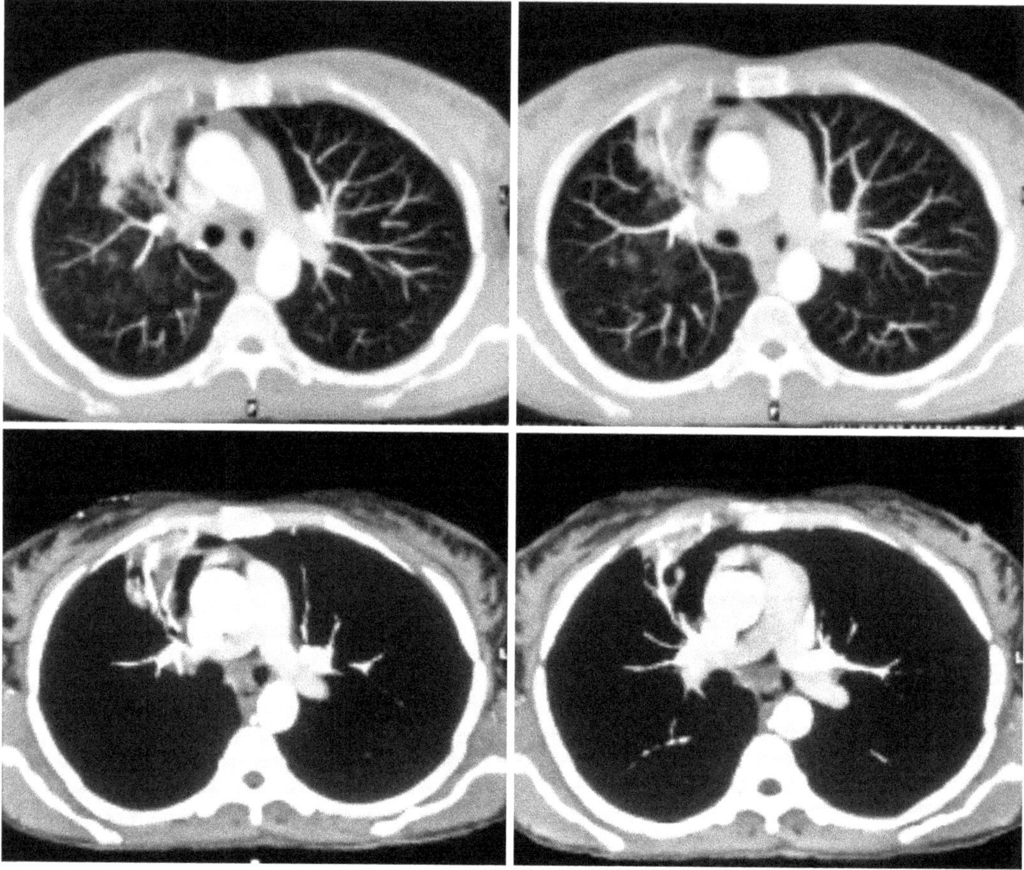

- *Description*: Focal dilatation of one of the pulmonary segmental artery (pseudoaneurysm) adjacent to tuberculous cavity.
- *Differential diagnosis*:
  - Vasculitis
  - Mycotic aneurysm
  - Rasmussen's aneurysm
- *Final impression*: Rasmussen's aneurysm

COMPUTED TOMOGRAPHY THORAX 15

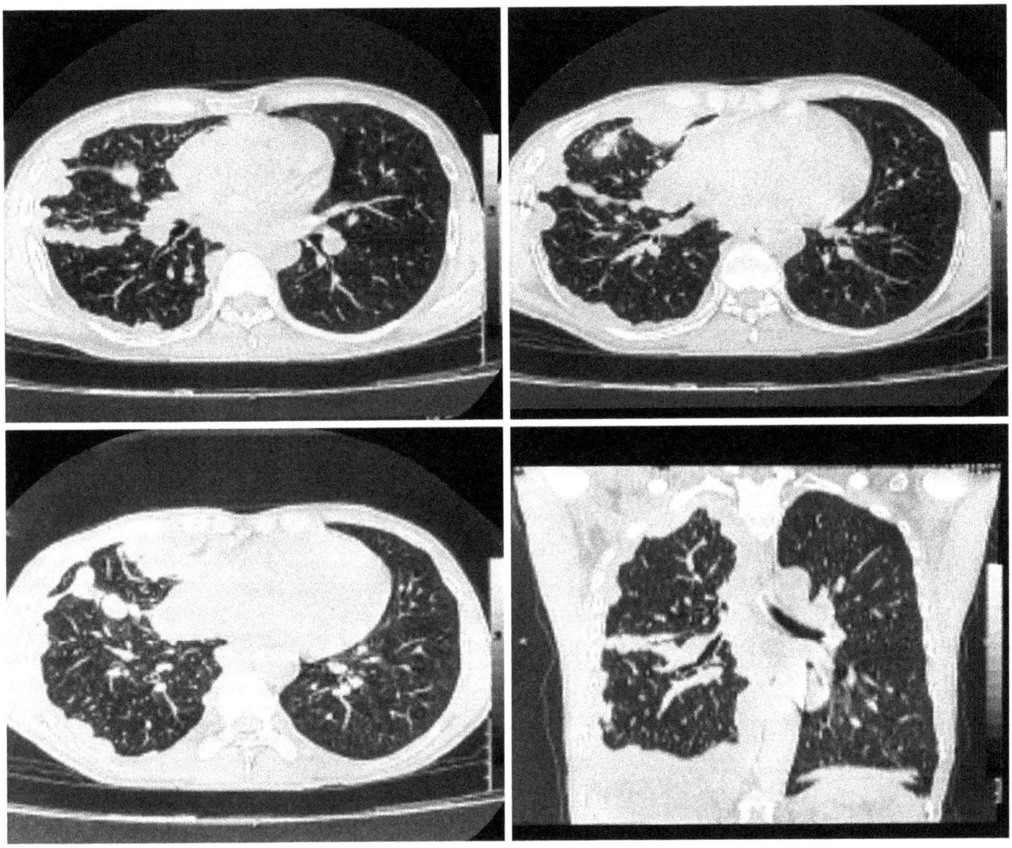

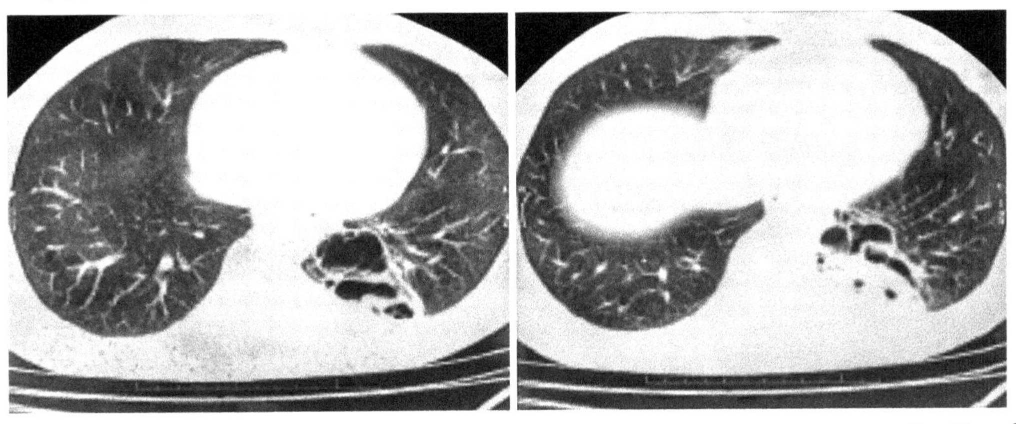

- *Description*: Nodules involving the transverse fissure, oblique fissure, and diaphragmatic pleura with pleural based lobulated lesion.
- *Final impression*: Right lung malignant mesothelioma with tumor extension into transverse and oblique fissure.

COMPUTED TOMOGRAPHY THORAX 16

Continued

Continued

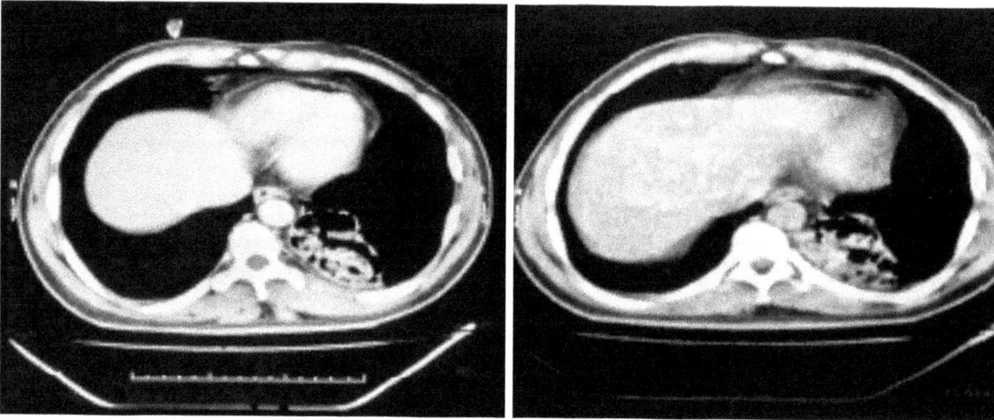

- *Description*: Left lower lobe multiple cavities
- *Differential diagnosis*:
  - Left lower lobe TB
  - Left lower lobe unresolved pneumonia
  - Left lower lobe bronchiectasis
  - Left sided congenital anomaly—sequestration
- *Final impression*: Left lung sequestration—confirmed by CT pulmonary angiography (CTPA).

▇ COMPUTED TOMOGRAPHY THORAX 17

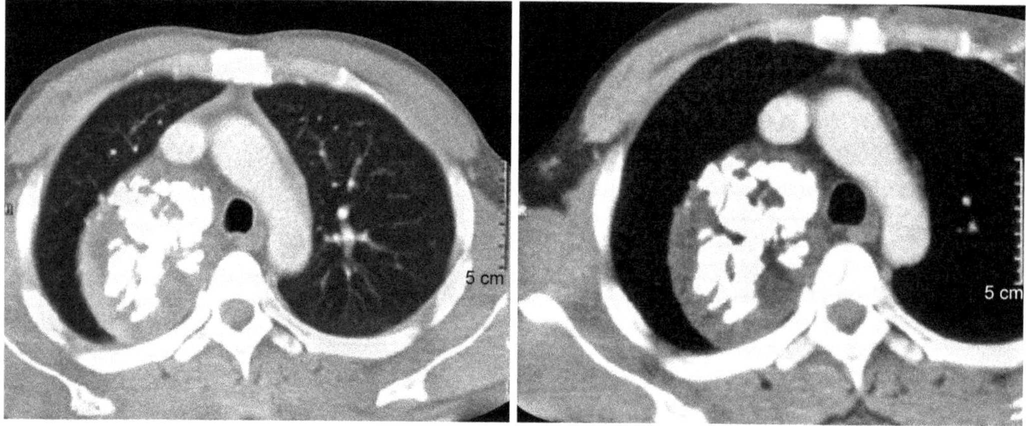

- *Description*: Dense calcified opacity inside right upper lobe soft tissue mass.
- *Differential diagnosis*:
  - Hamartoma
  - Schwannoma
- *Final impression*: Schwannoma—biopsy proven.

■ COMPUTED TOMOGRAPHY THORAX 18

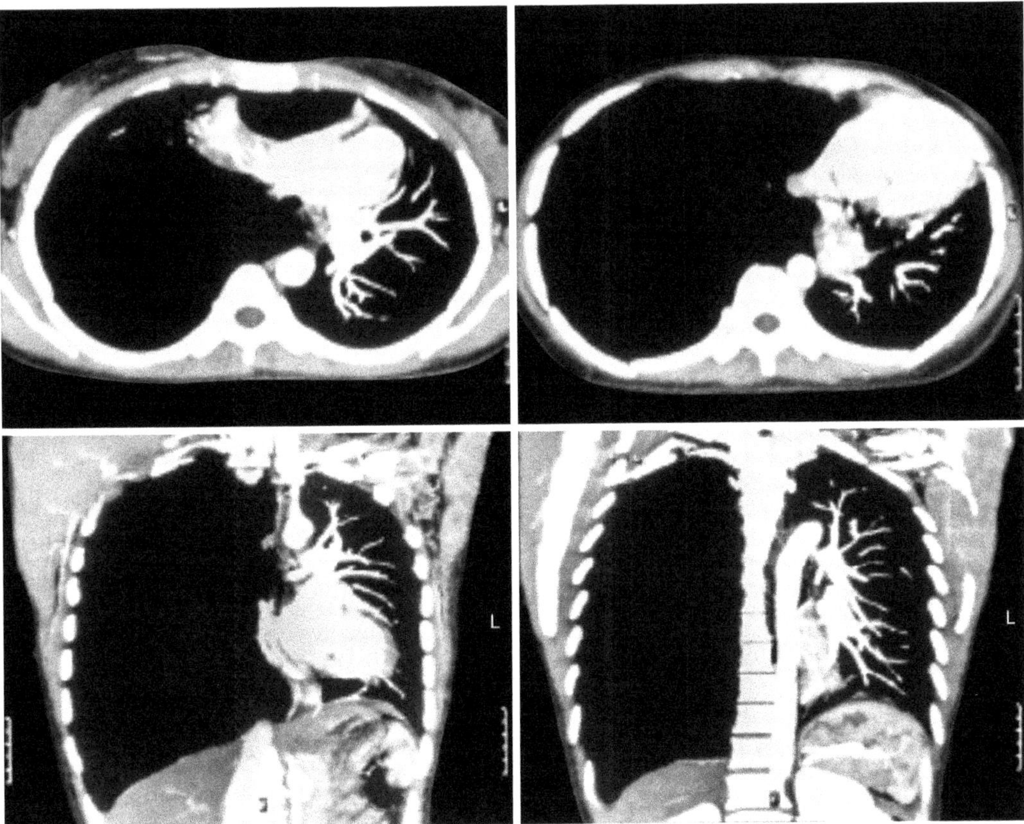

- *Description*: Hypertranslucency of right lung with herniation into left lung with absent bronchovascular marking on right side as seen on CTPA.
- *Differential diagnosis*:
  - Congenital lobar overinflation
  - Unilateral absence or proximal interruption of main pulmonary artery
  - Hypogenetic lung syndrome
  - MacLeod syndrome
- *Final impression*: MacLeods syndrome

USG Thorax

Susmita Kundu

INTRODUCTION

Ultrasound or ultrasonography (USG) is a medical imaging technique that uses high frequency sound waves and their echo. Ultrasound examination is a valuable method in the diagnosis of various pulmonary conditions including pleural disorders. It gives a real-time response characteristic and multiplanar imaging capability. Because of its portability, ultrasound is very important for examining patients at emergency unit and intensive care unit (ICU). Moreover, there is no radiation exposure to the patient.

BASIC PRINCIPLE

Sound is a form of energy transmitted through a medium. Ultrasound is defined as any sound with a frequency of >20 KHz, and for medical imaging it lies between 2 and 20 MHz.

Ultrasonography is based on the principle of emission of ultrasound waves and analysis of the echo thus generated. The ultrasound machine transmits high frequency sound pulses into the body using various probes and the sound waves travel into the body and hit a boundary between tissues. These sound waves reflect back to the probe from the patient as an echo and are relayed to the machine. The machine calculates the distance from the probe to the tissue or organ and displays the distance and intensities of the echoes on the screen forming a two-dimensional (2D) image.

APPLIED PHYSICS OF THORACIC ULTRASOUND

Ultrasound is based on two phenomenon:
1. Piezo-electrical
2. Acoustic impedance

Piezo-electric

Electricity causes the Piezo-electric crystal to bend/vibrate, thereby transducing the electric energy to sound energy (**Flowchart 1**).

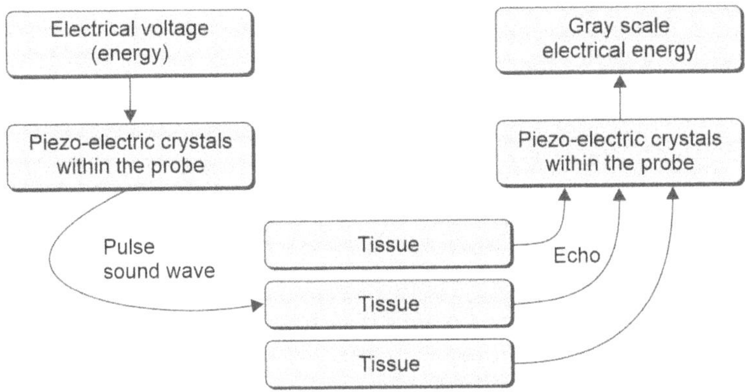

FLOWCHART 1: The Piezo-electric phenomenon.

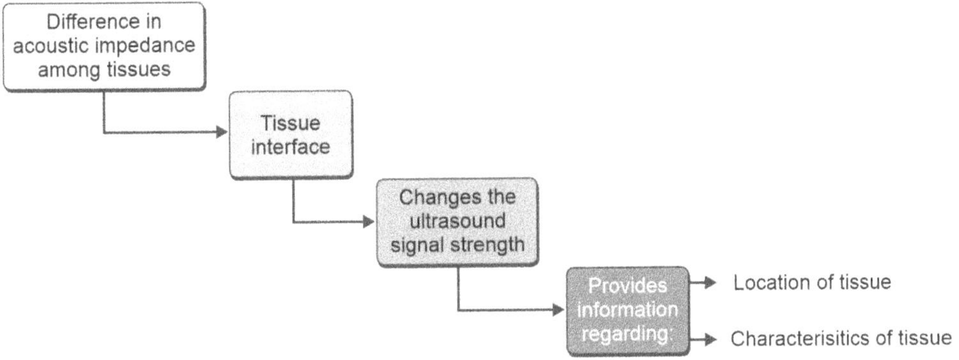

FLOWCHART 2: Mechanism of acoustic impedance.

Source: Processed into grayscale images on which ultrasound technology is based. Anantham and Ernst, 2010.

Acoustic Impedance

A *tissue interface* is formed where a tissue of one type abuts into another. These tissue are said to have different acoustic impedance. At a tissue interface ultrasound wave can be reflected or scattered **(Flowchart 2)**.

▨ USES OF THORACIC ULTRASOUND

Imaging

- *Pleural USG*:
  - Pleural effusion
  - Pneumothorax
  - Pleural thickening
- *Lung USG*:
  - Interstitial and alveolar edema
  - Consolidation

- ○ Lung mass and abscess
- ○ Atelectasis
- Thoracic ultrasound in respiratory failure
- Assessment of diaphragmatic function
- Monitoring the response to intervention

Interventional Procedures

- *Interventional procedures of the pleural space*:
  - ○ Thoracocentesis and catheter drainage
  - ○ Pleural biopsy
- *Pulmonary interventional procedures*:
  - ○ USG-guided lung biopsy
  - ○ Drainage of lung abscess
- *Mediastinal interventions*: Biopsy of large mediastinal mass or lymph nodes
- *Chest wall intervention*: Biopsy of chest wall mass

CONTRAINDICATIONS TO ULTRASOUND-GUIDED INTERVENTIONS

- *Absolute*:
  - ○ International normalized ratio (INR) >1.8
  - ○ Prothrombin time >50 seconds
  - ○ Platelet count <50,000
  - ○ Uncooperative patient
  - ○ Inability to maintain optimum position
  - ○ Inability to control coughing
- *Relative*:
  - ○ Bullous pulmonary emphysema
  - ○ Pulmonary hypertension

Complications

- Rate of pneumothorax is 2.8%.
- Hemorrhage or hemoptysis is observed in 0–2%.
- Tumor dissemination through the procedure of puncture is very rare (<0.003%).
- Air embolism (very rare)
- Perforation of other organs (uncommon).

Advantages

- Fast availability
- Bedside application
- Low rate of complications
- Absence of radiation exposure
- Low cost

Disadvantages

- Risks of complications with interventions
- Space occupying mass is hardly or not at all visible percutaneously.

ULTRASOUND SCANNERS

- Transmitter
- Transducer
- Receiver
- Processor
- Display
- Storage

Transmitter

Works on Piezo-electric effect. Ultrasound machine uses time elapsed with a presumed velocity (1,540 m/s) to calculate the depth of tissue interface. Image accuracy is therefore dependent on accuracy of presumed velocity.

Transducer/Probes

Ultrasound scanners emit and receive energy as waves to form pictures. Ultrasound transducer acts both as a speaker and a microphone—emits very short sound pulse and listens for returning echoes.

Transducer/probes are of the following types:
- *Sector scanner*: Fan-shaped beam. Requires a small surface for contact. Used in cardiac imaging.
- *Linear scanner*: Rectangular beam. A large contact area is required.
- *Curvilinear scanner*: Smaller scan head. Wider field of view.

Probe Position

- Sagittal
- Hold in pen holding fashion
- By the dominant hand
- Right angles to the ribs
- Make sure the landmarks (rib shadow) are in view.

ULTRASOUND MODES (FIGS. 1 AND 2)

- *A mode (amplitude):* A mode is used when precise depth and length measurement are needed. Amplitude of energy shown as peaks/waves. Used in ophthalmology.
- *B mode (brightness):* The amplitude of energy is shown as dots of varying intensity which allows conventional 2D image.
- *M mode (motion):* Image of a given object is monitored over time. These are moving 1D images. Used to see valves, vessels, and chambers.
- *D mode:* Doppler mode.

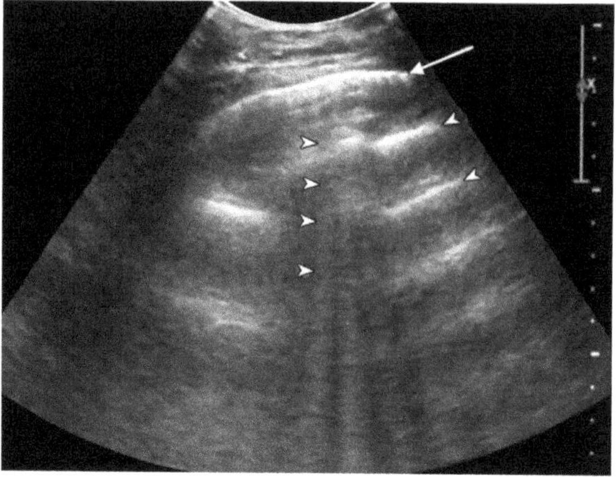

FIG. 1: B mode on ultrasonography (USG). US image shows A lines (large arrowheads) and B lines (small arrowheads). B lines are vertical hyperechoic artifacts originating from the pleural line (arrow) that extend to the edge of the screen and erase the A lines.

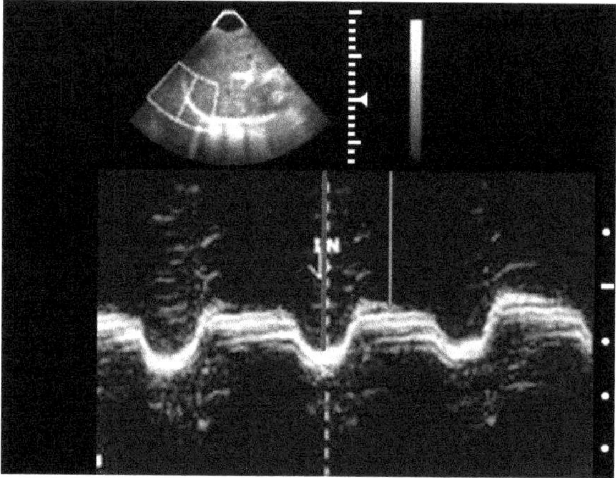

FIG. 2: M mode on ultrasonography (USG) showing normal diaphragmatic motion.

IMAGE PROPERTIES (FIG. 3)

- *Echogenicity*: Amount of energy reflected back from tissue interface.
- *Hyperechoic*: Greatest intensity—seen as white.
- *Anechoic*: No signal—seen as black.
- *Hypoechoic*: Intermediate—seen as gray.

ULTRASOUND ARTIFACTS

- Acoustic enhancement
- Acoustic shadowing
- Lateral cystic shadowing (edge artifact)

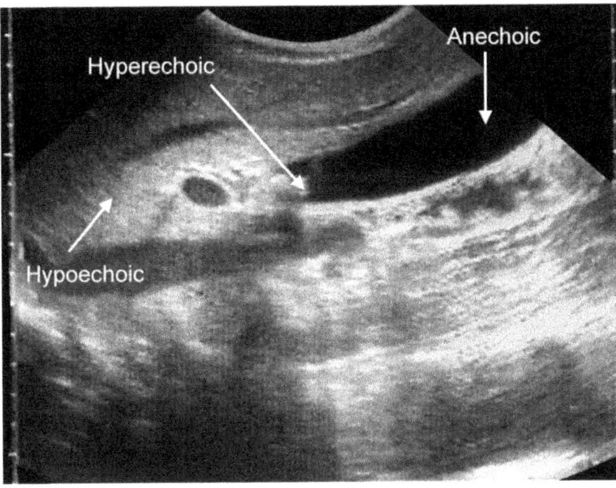

FIG. 3: Different types of image properties shown on ultrasonography (USG).

- Wide beam artifact
- Side lobe artifact
- Reverberation artifact
- Gain artifact
- Contact artifact

Acoustic Shadowing

- Occurs distal to any highly reflective or highly attenuating surface.
- Anechoic region lies behind bony structures.
- Shadow may be more prominent than the object causing it.

Acoustic Enhancement

- Opposite of acoustic shadow.
- Hyperechoic region located distal to fluid collection.
- Better ultrasound transmission allows enhancement of the ultrasound signal distal to the region.

Reverberation Artifact

- Several types
- Alternate white and dark lines
- Caused by the echo bouncing back and forth between two or more highly reflective surface.
- On the monitor parallel bands of reverbation echoes are seen.
- This causes a *comet tail pattern* **(Fig. 4)**.

BLUE POINT AND PLAPS POINT

- Upper bedside lung ultrasound in emergency (BLUE) point—upper lobe
- Lower BLUE point—middle lobe/lingula
- PLAPS (posterior or lateral alveolar and/or pleural syndrome point)—lower lobe

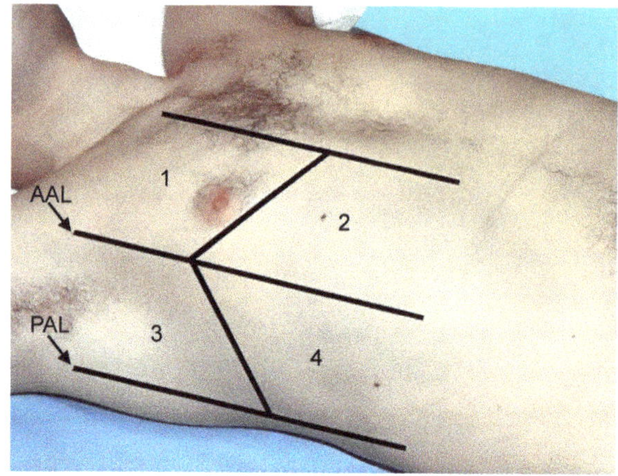

FIG. 4: Division of chest into four ultrasound zones on each side.
(AAL: anterior axillary line; PAL: posterior axillary line)

PLAPS Point

Stands for posterolateral alveolar/pleural syndrome.
- Posterolateral—round the back
- Alveolar—consolidation
- Pleural syndrome—pleural fluid
- The PLAPS point is the lowest point of the lung—the Morrison's pouch of the thorax.
- This is where we find all free effusions regardless of the volume.
- It is the posterior continuation of the lower BLUE point.

RIBS AND PLEURAL LINES

- Ribs are identified by the posterior acoustic shadowing which precludes the visualization of the deeper structures **(Fig. 5)**.
- Approximately, 0.5 cm below the rib line, a light hyperechoic horizontal line is seen—pleural line.
- Pleural line is the interface between soft tissues of chest wall and the aerated lung.
- During respiration, the two pleural surfaces slide against each other (air displacement) and appears as a shimmering white line.

ARTIFACTS

- Air in normal aerated lung stops progression of the ultrasound beam and hence the ultrasound image of the lung is composed of artifacts.
- These air artifacts arises from the pleural line.

Types of Artifacts

- *A lines* **(Fig. 6):**
  - Horizontal, hyperechoic, and static lines

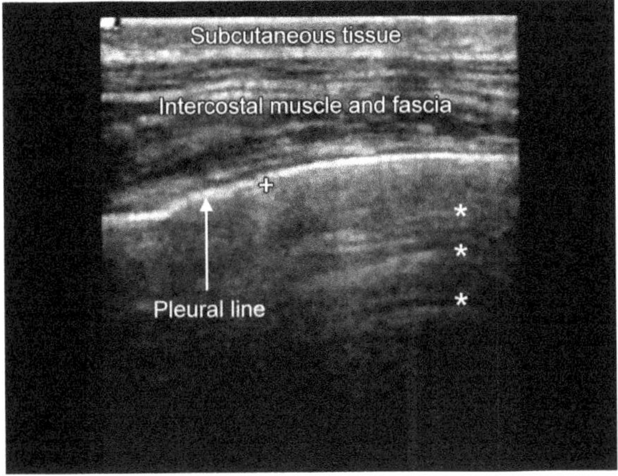

FIG. 5: Pleural line seen on B mode.

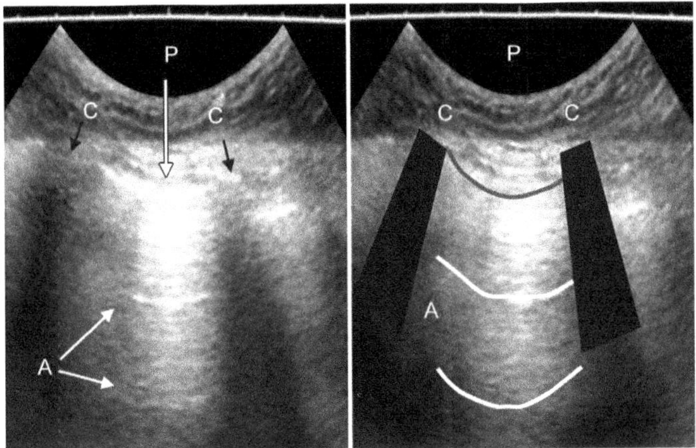

FIG. 6: A lines on ultrasonography (USG). Note the A lines (horizontal and light, indicated by letter A), pleural line (indicated by letter P), and ribs (indicated by letter C). In the figure on the right, the findings are illustrated.
Source: Dexheimer Neto et al., 2012.

- Repeat at regular intervals
- Decay with depth
- Obliterated by B lines
- They are reverberation artifacts from pleura
- Seen in two-thirds of normal lung and pneumothorax
- *B lines*
  - Hyperechoic, vertical lines
  - Originates from the pleural line
  - Moves with respiration
  - Reaches base of the screen
  - Obliterates A lines
  - More than two B lines at a time is abnormal

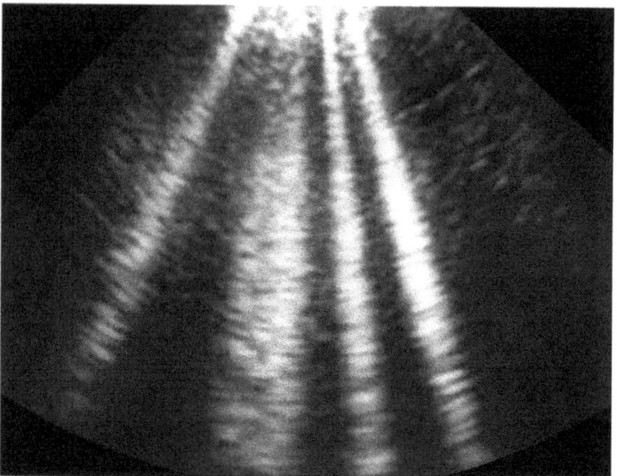

FIG. 7: B lines on ultrasonography (USG).

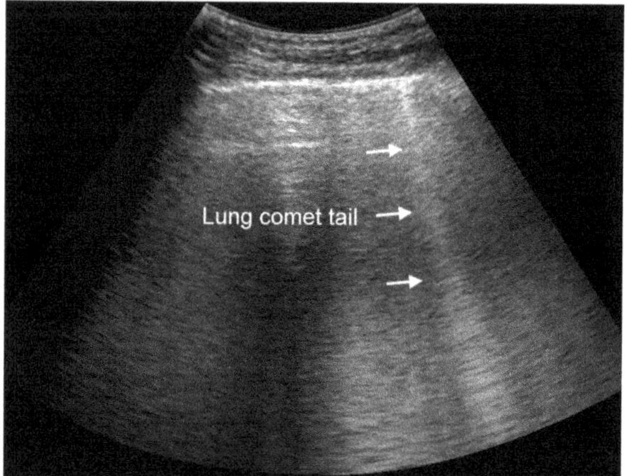

FIG. 8: Lung comet tail on ultrasonography (USG) thorax.

- ○ Equivalent to Kerley's B-line
- ○ Implies air/fluid mix, a interlobular septa **(Fig. 7)**

Comet Tail Artifacts

Defined as a hyperechogenic, coherent bundle with a narrow base spreading from the transducer to the further border of the screen. It extends to the edge of the screen and arises only from the pleural line. These are also called by the descriptive "comet tail artifacts" **(Fig. 8)**.

Lung Rockets

- When several B lines are visible in a single scan, the pattern resembles a rocket, a lift-off, this is called lung rockets.
- Three or more B lines per lung field—lung rockets
- Up to one-third of normal patients have rockets in the dependent region.
- So rockets in PLAPS point does not matter **(Fig. 9)**.

Importance of Lung Rockets
- In all windows—cardiogenic pulmonary edema
- Patchy with spread areas—noncardiogenic pulmonary edema
- Localized—pneumonia/chronic interstitial diseases like fibrosis
- In the base—normal
- *Z lines* **(Fig. 10)**
    - Ill-defined vertical lines arising from the pleura
    - Not reaching the distal end of the screen
    - Does not move with respiration
    - Does not obliterate the A lines
    - Seen in normal persons as well as in pneumothorax
- *E lines:* Comet tail artifacts can be seen superficial to the pleural line in those with parietal emphysema or parietal echogenic multiple foreign bodies (shot gun pellets). These are called E lines.

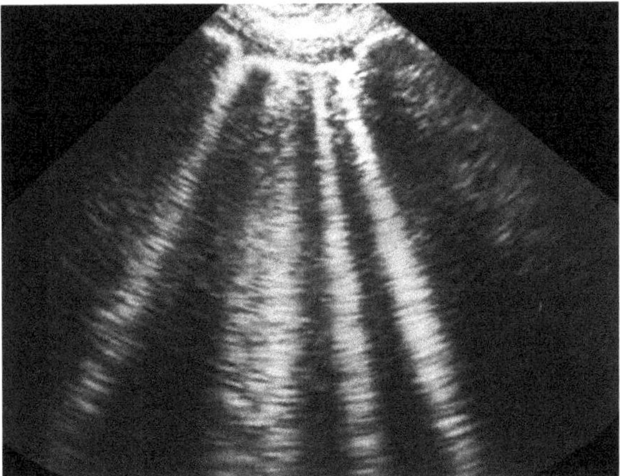

FIG. 9: Lung rockets.

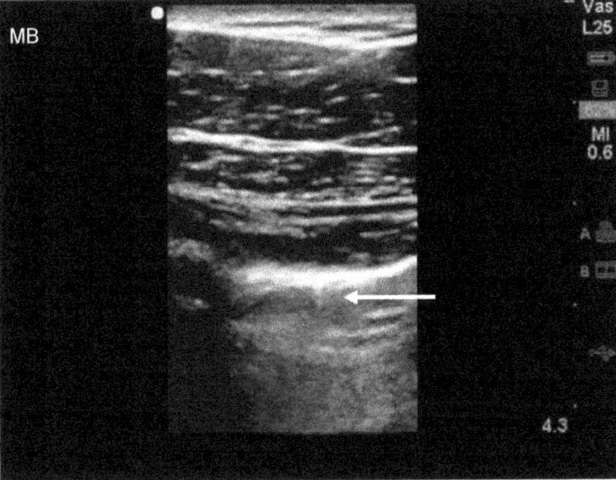

FIG. 10: Z lines.

LUNG SLIDING

- Visceral pleura glides over the parietal pleura in regular cycles.
- Seen on B mode of USG.

Importance

- A lines + sliding—normal dry lung
- A lines without sliding—pneumothorax
- Rockets + sliding— apolipoprotein (APO)-b profile
- Rockets without sliding—acute respiratory distress syndrome (ARDS)/pneumonia B' profile

Seashore sign: The image best seen in an M mode as the superficial parietal layers, are motionless and have a horizontal pattern of lines, while the area deep to the pleural line appears "granular" as the motion of the pleural line is reflected all over this area **(Fig. 11)**.

DIAPHRAGM

It appears as:
- Thin
- Curvilinear
- Echogenic
- Moves with respiration
- Moves caudally with respiration **(Fig. 12)**

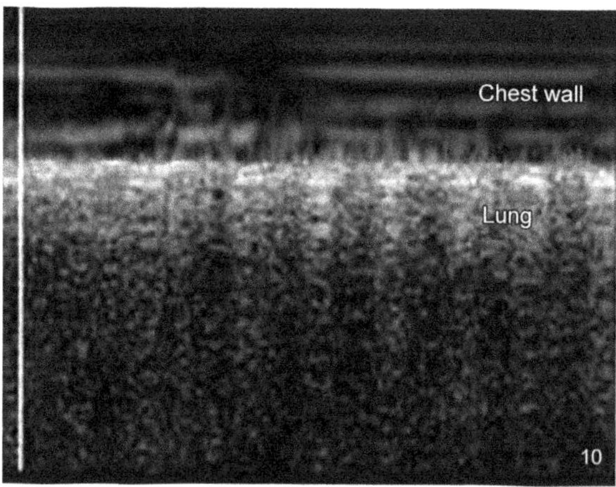

FIG. 11: Seashore sign. Lung sliding is easily identified on B mode US; on M mode US, lung sliding appears as a specific sign, known as the Seashore sign, which is characterized by a *Linear pattern-corresponding* to the chest wall (no movement)-above the pleural line and a *homogeneous granular pattern*—an artifact generated by respiratory cycles and air movement below the pleural line.

Source: Anantham and Ernst, 2010.

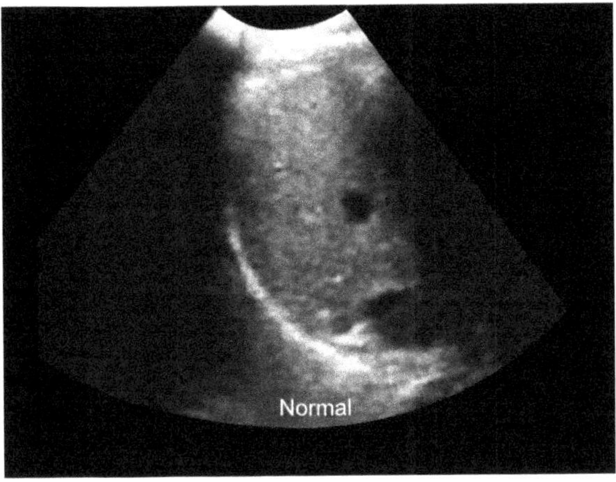

FIG. 12: A normal diaphragm on B mode of ultrasonography (USG).

INTERPRETATIONS

Normal Lung

- A profile
- Up to two B lines per window
- PLAPS negative
- Seashore sign on M mode

Pneumothorax

- A' profile
- Absent lung sliding
- Absence of B lines on the same side
- Loss of comet tail artifacts
- Exaggerated horizontal artifacts
- Absent lung rockets
- Lung point sign unless lung is completely collapsed
- Absent lung impulse
- Broadening of pleural line to a band
- M mode—Barcode sign or stratosphere sign

Stratosphere Sign

The sign is an imaging finding using a 3.5–7.5 MHz ultrasound probe in the 4th and 5th intercostal spaces in the anterior clavicular line using the M mode of the machine. This finding is seen in the M mode tracing as pleura, and lung being indistinguishable as linear hyperechogenic lines, and is fairly reliable for diagnosis of a pneumothorax. Even though the stratospheric sign can be an indication of pneumothorax, its absence is not at all reliable to rule out pneumothorax as definitive diagnosis usually requires X-ray or computed tomography (CT) of thorax **(Fig. 13)**.

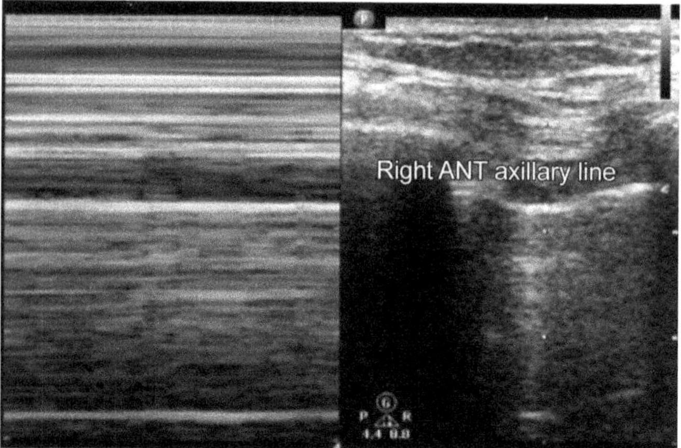

FIG. 13: Stratosphere sign seen on M mode.

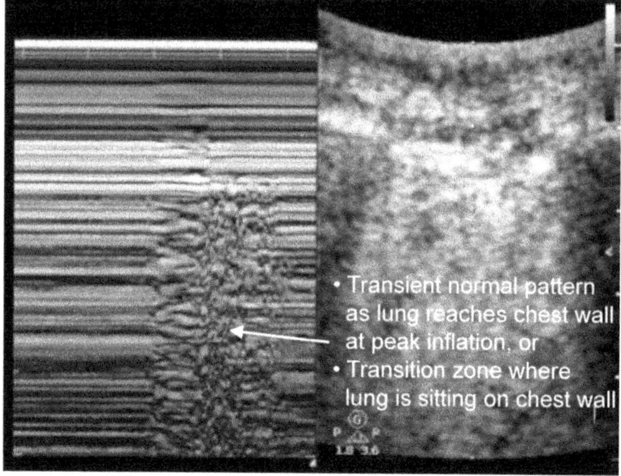

FIG. 14: Lung point sign (on M mode) seen in pneumothorax.

LUNG POINT SIGN

- Highly specific for pneumothorax
- It involves visualizing the point where the visceral pleura begins to separate from the parietal pleura at the margin of the pneumothorax.
- The junction between sliding lung and absent sliding is known as lung point.
- It is 100% specific for pneumothorax and also gives an indication about the size of the pneumothorax by its location **(Fig. 14)**.

PLEURAL EFFUSION

- Appears as a hypoechoic (dark) and homogeneous structure in the dependent parts of the lung.
- Present both in inspiration and expiration.

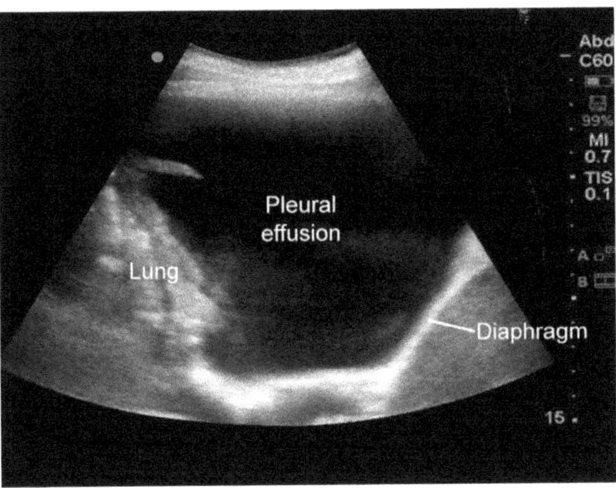

FIG. 15: Pleural effusion seen on B mode.

Signs Seen in Pleural Effusion (Fig. 15)

- Curtain sign
- Sinusoid sign
- Gator sign
- Plankton sign
- Quad sign
- Jelly fish sign
- Hematocrit sign
- Heterogeneously echogenic collection
- Swirling debris
- Hematocrit sign
- Pleural thickening >10 mm
- Diaphragmatic thickening >7 mm
- Presence of pleural nodules

COMPLICATED PARAPNEUMONIC EFFUSION/EMPYEMA (FIG. 16)

- Heterogeneously echogenic collection
- Presence of septations
- Hematocrit sign

Nature of Pleural Effusion

- Fibrin strands swimming in the fluid with undulations, debris, or loculation suggest pus or blood.
- Other than this, the nature of the pleural fluid cannot be accurately determined on USG thorax.

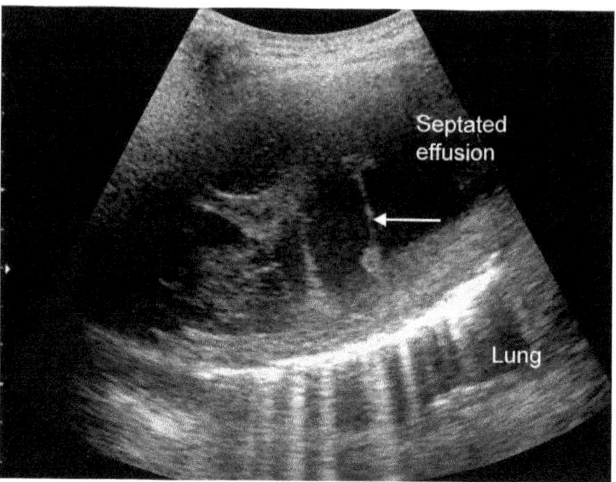

FIG. 16: Septated pleural effusion.

Volume Estimation of Pleural Effusion

- It is difficult to measure the volume of pleural fluid accurately with ultrasound.
- If the depth of the fluid is >5 cm, then it is likely there is >500 mL of pleural fluid.
- The amount of pleural fluid can be estimated by the following formula:

$$V \text{ (mL)} = 20 \times \text{Sep}$$

Where, V—volume, Sep—maximal distance between the 2 pleural layers (visceral and parietal pleura).

Sinusoid Sign

M mode finding indicating presence of pleural effusion. Due to the cyclical movement of the lung in inspiration and expiration, the motion-time tracing (M mode) ultrasound shows a sinusoid appearance between the fluid and the line tissue. This finding indicates possibly but not with certainty, of a pleural effusion, empyema, and blood in pleural space (hemothorax).

Curtain Sign

B mode finding showing intermittent appearance of lung expanding into pleural effusion.

Quad Sign

A pleural effusion has an anechoic appearance often delineated by the pleural line, the rib shadows, and the lung line, called the quad sign.

Plankton Sign

An anechoic fluid collection is often a transudative effusion, whereas a heterogeneous fluid collection is typically an exudative effusion. Dynamic swirling debris commonly seen in exudative effusions is called the plankton sign.

Hematocrit Sign

Highly cellular effusions may appear on static imaging as layered as cells collect in a dependent fashion by gravity, termed the hematocrit sign **(Fig. 17)**.

Jelly Fish Sign

With large pleural effusions, one may identify compressed, airless lung floating within the effusion, termed the jelly fish sign **(Fig. 18)**.

PNEUMONIA

- Hyperechoic consolidated area of varying size and shape with irregular borders.
- Echotexture can appear homogeneous or inhomogeneous.

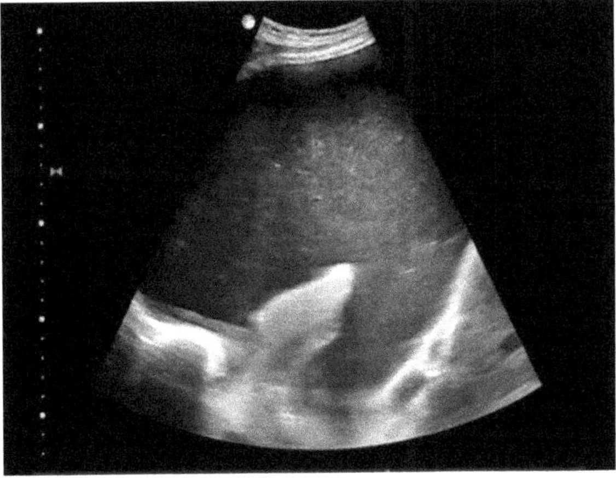

FIG. 17: Hematocrit sign.

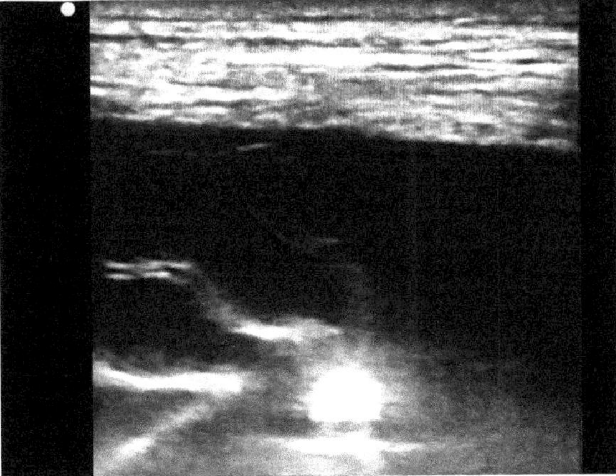

FIG. 18: Jelly fish sign.

- *Most common features*: Air bronchogram which is characterized by lens-shape internal echoes within the hypodense area or echogenic lines and corresponds to air-filled bronchioles and bronchi.
- Liver like in the early stage
- Lenticular air trapping
- Blurred and serrated margins
- Reverberation echoes in the margin
- Presence of A/B profile, C profile, or B' profile
- PLAPS positive
- Fluid bronchogram **(Fig. 19)**

DIAPHRAGMATIC PARALYSIS

- Diaphragm moving <5 mm or paradoxically in inspiration
- Loss of normal thickening during inspiration
- Loss of lung sliding sign
- Normal diaphragm thickens on inspiration end-inspiratory thickness 20% or more above baseline **(Fig. 20)**.

USE OF ULTRASOUND IN INTERVENTIONAL PROCEDURES

BLUES Protocol

- The A profile associates anterior lung sliding with A lines.
- The A' profile is an A profile with abolished lung sliding.
- The B profile associates anterior lung sliding with lung rockets.

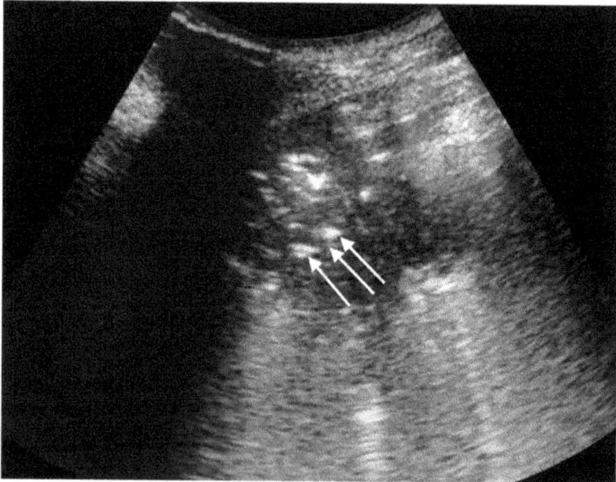

FIG. 19: Air bronchogram seen in pneumonia. Posterior intercostal scan shows a hypoechoic consolidated area that contains multiple echogenic lines that represent an air bronchogram.

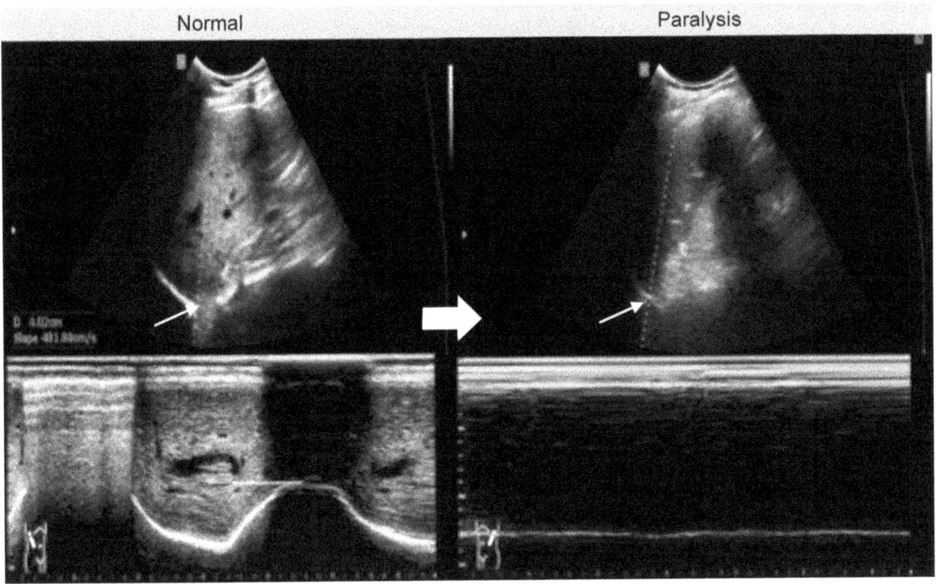

FIG. 20: Diaphragmatic paralysis.

- The B′ profile is a B profile with abolished lung sliding.
- The C profile indicates anterior lung consolidation, regardless of size and number. A thickened, irregular pleural line is an equivalent.
- The A/B profile is a half A profile at one lung, a half B profile at another.
- The PLAPS profile designates posterolateral alveolar and/or pleural syndrome. PLAPS are sought for after detection of an A profile (a pattern compatible with pulmonary embolism) and of a free venous network (a pattern making the diagnosis of embolism less likely). The profile combining A profile, free veins, and PLAPS is called A-V-PLAPS-profile.

Other Protocols

- *FALLS (fluid administration limited by lung sonography) protocol*: For substantial pericardial effusion (likened to pericardial tamponade in acute circulatory failure), then for right ventricle dilatation (suggesting pulmonary embolism) **(Flowchart 3)**.
- *SESAME protocol*: A fast protocol devoted to cardiac arrest, assesses the lung before the heart.
- *PINK protocol*: ARDS.

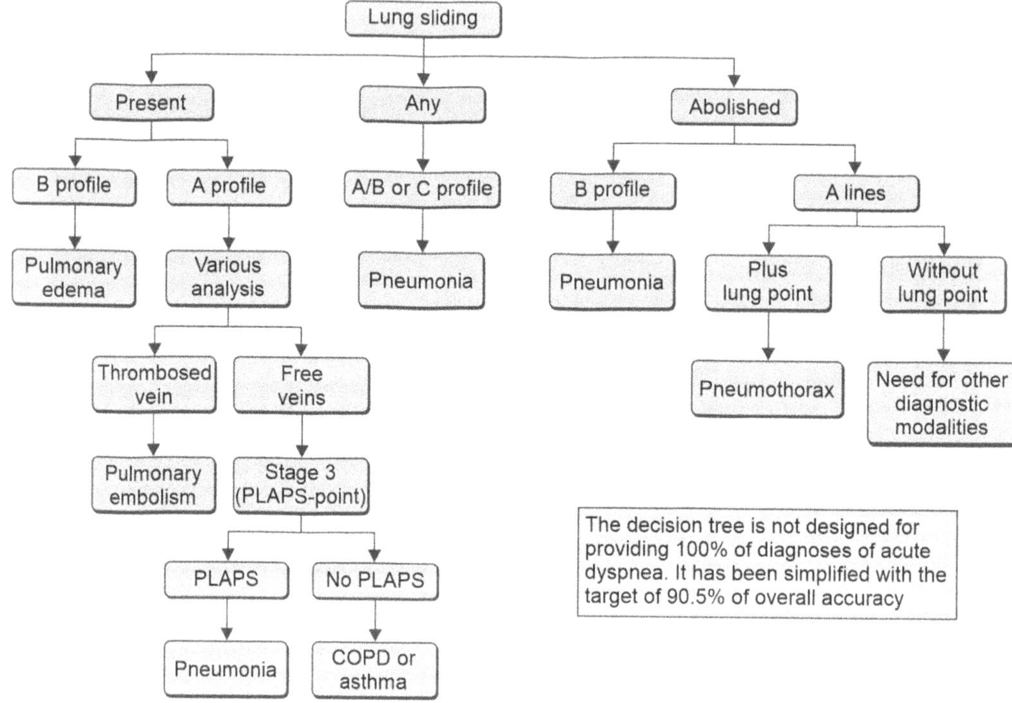

FLOWCHART 3: BLUE protocol.

Note: A profile means predominantly A lines. B profile means predominantly multiple anterior diffuse B lines. A/B profile means predominant A lines on one side and predominant B lines on the other side. C profile means anterior alveolar consolidation(s). PLAPS means posterolateral alveolar and/or pleural syndrome detected on a lateral subposterior sonological examination.

(BLUE: bedside lung ultrasound in emergency; COPD: chronic obstructive pulmonary disease).

Source: Figure taken from ERS.

Arterial Blood Gas Analysis

Susmita Kundu, Arya Chaudhuri

INTRODUCTION

Respiratory acid base disorders are commonly seen in the intensive care unit and patients admitted with acute exacerbation of chronic obstructive pulmonary disease (AECOPD) with respiratory failure, acute severe asthma, and acute respiratory distress syndrome (ARDS). It can occur independently or coexist with metabolic acid base disorders.

So every respiratory physician must have an overall knowledge of respiratory acid base disorders.

Acid base abnormalities and compensatory changes on the Henderson–Hasselbalch equation is shown in **Table 1**.

- pH = 7.36–7.44
- pCO_2 = 36–44 mmHg
- HCO_3^- = 22–26 mEq/L

To evaluate mixed acid base disorders if you remember the following things, it will be easy to interpret:

- *Primary metabolic acidosis*:
    - Expected pCO_2 = (HCO_3^-) + 15 mmHg
- *Primary metabolic alkalosis*:
    - Expected pCO_2 = (HCO_3^-) + 15 mmHg (less sensitive)

TABLE 1: Acid base abnormalities and compensatory changes.		
Disorder	**Primary change**	**Compensatory response**
Metabolic acidosis	$\downarrow HCO_3^-$	$\downarrow CO_2$
Metabolic alkalosis	$\uparrow HCO_3^-$	$\uparrow CO_2$
Respiratory acidosis	$\uparrow CO_2$	$\uparrow HCO_3^-$
Respiratory alkalosis	$\downarrow CO_2$	$\downarrow HCO_3^-$

- *Primary respiratory acidosis*:
    - HCO_3^- is increased by 1 mm/L for every 10 mm Hg increase in pCO_2 above 40 mmHg (in acute condition).
    - HCO_3^- is increased by 3 mm/L for every 10 mm Hg increase in pCO_2 above 40 mm Hg (in chronic condition).
- *Primary respiratory alkalosis*:
    - HCO_3^- is ↓ by 2 mm/L for every 10 mm Hg ↓ in pCO_2 (in acute condition).
    - HCO_3^- is ↓ by 4–5 mm/L for every 10 mm Hg ↓ in pCO_2 (in chronic condition).
- *Anion GAP*:
    - $(Na + K) - (Cl + HCO_3) = UA - UC$ = anion gap; *or*
    - $Na - (Cl + HCO_3) = UA\text{-}UC$ = anion gap
    - UA = unmeasured anion (-ve change)
    - UC = unmeasured cation (+ve changed)

Albumin is a major unmeasured anion in serum and hypoalbuminemia and will therefore lead to the determination of a falsely low anion gap.

- Corrected anion gap = CAG
- CAG = anion gap + 2.5 [normal albumin (g/dL) – measured albumin (g/dL)]
- Normal anion gap is between 8 and 12 mEq/L
- Example of one arterial blood gas (ABG)
    - pH—7.11
    - pCO_2—76.7
    - pO_2—96.7
    - Na^+—115
    - K^+—5.9
    - Cl—70
    - HCO_3—23.8

In this patient, anion gap = $(115 + 5.9) - (23.8 + 70) = 27.1$

So, this is a case of respiratory acidosis with high anion gap metabolic acidosis, and as K^+ is high, this patient is probably suffering from chronic kidney disease.

ARTERIAL BLOOD GAS 1

```
            OPTI Medical OPTI CCA
              Patient Report


     Pat. ID:55
     Sample No.:950

     ACID/BASE 37.0°C
       pH      7.31
       PCO2↓    23      mmHg
       PO2     154      mmHg
       BE      -13.5    mmol/L
       tCO2     12.0    mmol/L
       HCO3     11.3    mmol/L
       BB       31.6    mmol/L
       BEact   -13.3    mmol/L
       BEecf   -15.0    mmol/L
       stHCO3   13.7    mmol/L
       st.pH    7.159
       cH+      49.4    nmol/L

     ELECTROLYTES
       Na+     136      mmol/L
       K+  ↓    3.2     mmol/L
       Ca++↓  0.54      mmol/L
       nCa++   0.52     mmol/L

     HEMOGLOBIN/OXYGEN STATUS
       tHb ↓   8.2      g/dL
       SO2      99      %
       Hct(c)   25      %
       SO2(c)   99      %
       AaDO2    44.5    mmHg
       O2Ct     11.7    vol%
       P50(c)  -----    mmHg

     ENTERED PARAMETERS
       Temp  37.0       °C
       Sex Female
       Hb Type Adult
       MCHC   33.3      %
       FIO2   0.32
       RQ  0.84
       P50   26.7       mmHg

     Barometer:747.9 mmHg
     Operator ID:
     S/N:9851  LOT:516400


     (Ref.Lim)
       pH      7.20 -   7.60
       PCO2      30 -     50 mmHg
       PO2       70 -    700 mmHg
       Na+      135 -    145 mmol/L
       K+       3.5 -    5.1 mmol/L
       Ca++    1.12 -   1.32 mmol/L
       tHb     12.0 -   17.0 g/dL
       SO2       90 -    100 %

     MESSAGES
       PCO2 under    30 (Ref.Lim)
       K+   under   3.5 (Ref.Lim)
       Ca++ under  1.12 (Ref.Lim)
       tHb  under  12.0 (Ref.Lim)
```

- PH—7.31
- PCO_2—23
- PO_2—154
- NA—136
- K—3.2
- HCO_3—11.3

- *Interpretation*: Metabolic acidosis—PH, HCO_3, PCO_2
- *Causes of metabolic acidosis*:
  - Diabetic ketoacidosis
  - Lactic acidosis
  - Renal failure
  - Ethanol poisoning
  - Gastrointestinal (GI) bicarbonate loss

ARTERIAL BLOOD GAS 2

```
Results: Gases+
pH        7.129          Low
pCO2      100.5   mmHg   High
pO2       141.0   mmHg   High
cHCO3-    33.3    mmol/L High
BE(ecf)   4.1     mmol/L High
cSO2      97.9    %

Results: Chem+
Na+       144     mmol/L
K+        5.3     mmol/L High
Ca++      1.00    mmol/L Low
cTCO2     36.4    mmol/L High
Hct       32      %      Low
cHgb      10.8    g/dL   Low
BE(b)     1.9     mmol/L

Results: Meta+
Glu       122     mg/dL  High
Lac       0.67    mmol/L

Reference Ranges
pH         7.350 - 7.450
pCO2        35.0 - 48.0    mmHg
pO2         83.0 - 108.0   mmHg
cHCO3-      21.0 - 28.0    mmol/L
BE(ecf)     -2.0 - 3.0     mmol/L
cSO2        94.0 - 98.0    %
Na+          138 - 146     mmol/L
K+           3.5 - 4.5     mmol/L
Ca++        1.15 - 1.33    mmol/L
cTCO2       22.0 - 29.0    mmol/L
Hct           38 - 51      %
cHgb        12.0 - 17.0    g/dL
BE(b)       -2.0 - 3.0     mmol/L
Glu           74 - 100     mg/dL
Lac         0.56 - 1.39    mmol/L
```

- PH—7.129
- PCO_2—100.5
- PO_2—141
- HCO_3—33.3
- Na—144
- K—5.3

- *Interpretation*: Acute respiratory acidosis—↓↓PH, ↑↑PCO_2, ↑HCO_3
- *Causes of acute respiratory acidosis*:
  - Pulmonary cause
    - Type 2 respiratory failure in acute exacerbation of stable chronic obstructive pulmonary disease (COPD)
    - Occasionally in acute exacerbation of asthma
  - Central cause
    - Cerebrovascular accident (CVA)
    - Trauma
    - Drug induced
  - Neuromuscular
    - Poliomyelitis
    - Myasthenia gravis
    - Kyphoscoliosis
    - Myopathy

- ○ Miscelleneous
  - – Obesity
  - – Hypoventilation

ARTERIAL BLOOD GAS 3

```
ACID/BASE 37.0°C
  pH      7.35
  PCO2↑   64      mmHg
  PO2     91      mmHg
  BE       7.5    mmol/L
  tCO2    37.0    mmol/L
  HCO3    35.0    mmol/L
  BB      54.3    mmol/L
  BEact    7.7    mmol/L
  BEecf    9.5    mmol/L
  stHCO3  30.2    mmol/L
  st.pH   7.502
  cH+     44.4    nmol/L

ELECTROLYTES
  Na+     135     mmol/L
  K+       3.9    mmol/L
  Ca++↓   0.81    mmol/L
  nCa++    0.79   mmol/L

HEMOGLOBIN/OXYGEN STATUS
  tHb     12.1    g/dL
  SO2     97      %
  Hct(c)    36    %
  SO2(c)    97    %
  AaDO2  119.9    mmHg
  O2Ct    16.6    vol%
  P50(c)  27.9    mmHg

ENTERED PARAMETERS
  Temp 37.0     °C
  Sex Female
  Hb Type Adult
  MCHC  33.3    %
  FIO2  0.40
  RQ  0.84
  P50  26.7     mmHg

Barometer:752.7 mmHg
Operator ID:48
S/N:9851  LOT:516400


  (Ref.Lim)
  pH      7.20 -  7.60
  PCO2      30 -    50 mmHg
  PO2       70 -   700 mmHg
  Na+      135 -   145 mmol/L
  K+       3.5 -   5.1 mmol/L
  Ca++    1.12 -  1.32 mmol/L
  tHb     12.0 -  17.0 g/dL
  SO2       90 -   100 %

MESSAGES
  PCO2 over    50 (Ref.Lim)
  Ca++ under 1.12 (Ref.Lim)
```

- PH—7.35
- PCO_2—64
- PO_2—91
- HCO_3—35
- Na—135
- K—3.9

- *Interpretation*: Chronic respiratory acidosis—↓PH, ↑PCO_2, ↑HCO_3
- *Causes of chronic respiratory acidosis*:
  - ○ Advanced COPD
  - ○ Obesity hypoventilation syndrome

ARTERIAL BLOOD GAS 4

```
Pat. ID:03
Sample No.:3202

ACID/BASE 37.0°C
 pH     7.52
 PCO2↑   54      mmHg
 PO2    111      mmHg
 BE     18.6     mmol/L
 tCO2   45.2     mmol/L
 HCO3   43.5     mmol/L
 BB     64.1     mmol/L
 BEact  19.3     mmol/L
 BEecf  20.7     mmol/L
 stHCO3 40.8     mmol/L
 st.pH  7.633
 cH+    30.0     nmol/L

ELECTROLYTES
 Na+    138      mmol/L
 K+  ↓  2.5      mmol/L
 Ca++↓ 0.92      mmol/L
 nCa++  0.98     mmol/L

HEMOGLOBIN/OXYGEN STATUS
 tHb ↓  9.0      g/dL
 SO2    98       %
 Hct(c) 27       %
 SO2(c) 99       %
 AaDO2  51.9     mmHg
 O2Ct   12.7     vol%
 P50(c) 26.7     mmHg

ENTERED PARAMETERS
 Temp  37.0     °C
 Sex Male
 Hb Type Adult
 MCHC  33.3     %
 FIO2  0.32
 RQ    0.84
 P50   26.7     mmHg

Barometer:746.6 mmHg
Operator ID:
S/N:9851  LOT:552403


(Ref.Lim)
 pH     7.20 -   7.60
 PCO2    30 -     50 mmHg
 PO2     70 -    700 mmHg
 Na+    135 -    145 mmol/L
 K+     3.5 -    5.1 mmol/L
 Ca++  1.12 -   1.32 mmol/L
 tHb   12.0 -   17.0 g/dL
 SO2     90 -    100 %

MESSAGES
PCO2 over   50 (Ref.Lim)
K+   under  3.5 (Ref.Lim)
Ca++ under 1.12 (Ref.Lim)
tHb  under 12.0 (Ref.Lim)
```

- PH—7.52
- PCO_2—54
- PO_2—111
- HCO_3—43.5
- Na—138
- K—2.5

- *Interpretation*: Metabolic alkalosis due to hypokalemia—↑PH, ↑PCO_2, ↑↑HCO_3
- *Causes of metabolic alkalosis*:
  - Diarrhea
  - Vomiting
  - Drugs—diuretic, steroid
  - Exogenous bicarbonate load
  - Primary aldosteronism
  - Hypokalemia

ARTERIAL BLOOD GAS 5

```
ACID/BASE 37.0°C
  pH   ↓ 6.99
  PCO2↑   80      mmHg
  PO2    ·119     mmHg
  BE      -12.9    mmol/L
  tCO2    21.4    mmol/L
  HCO3    19.0    mmol/L
  BB      33.3    mmol/L
  BEact   -13.8    mmol/L
  BEecf   -12.4    mmol/L
  stHCO3  14.2    mmol/L
  st.pH   7.174
  cH+ ·   101.7    nmol/L

ELECTROLYTES
  Na+     142     mmol/L
  K+      3.5     mmol/L
  Ca++↓ 0.96     mmol/L
  nCa++   0.78     mmol/L

HEMOGLOBIN/OXYGEN STATUS
  tHb ↓ 10.5     g/dL
  SO2      94     %
  Hct(c)   32     %
  SO2(c)   94     %
  AaDO2   17 5    mmHg
  O2Ct    14 2    vol%
  P50(c)  - - -    mmHg

ENTERED PARAMETERS
  Temp   37.0    °C
  Sex Male
  Hb Type Adult
  MCHC   33.3    %
  FIO2   0.32
  RQ   0.84
  P50   26.7     mmHg

Barometer:755.7 mmHg
Operator ID:
S/N:9851   LOT:530403
```

- PH—6.99
- PCO$_2$—80
- PO$_2$—119
- HCO$_3$—19
- Na—142
- K—3.5

- *Interpretation*: Mixed acidosis—respiratory acidosis with metabolic acidosis ↓↓PH, ↑PCO$_2$, ↓HCO$_3$
- *Causes*:
    - AECOPD/Type 2 respiratory failure (T2rf) with sepsis
    - T2rf with diabetic ketoacidosis (DKA)
    - Postcardiac arrest status
    - Airway obstruction following polytrauma
    - T2rf with renal failure
- *Management*: Patient needs urgent mechanical ventilation with treatment of primary cause.

ARTERIAL BLOOD GAS 6

```
ACID/BASE 37.0°C
  pH     7.33
  PCO2   127      mmHg
  PO2    122      mmHg
  BE      32.4    mmol/L
  tCO2    68.9    mmol/L
  HCO3    65.0    mmol/L
  BB      78.8    mmol/L
  BEact   32.4    mmol/L
  BEecf   39.0    mmol/L
  stHCO3  57.4    mmol/L
  st.pH   7.781
  cH+     47.2    nmol/L

ELECTROLYTES
  Na+    142      mmol/L
  K+ ↓   2.6      mmol/L
  Ca++   1.12     mmol/L
  nCa++  1.08     mmol/L

HEMOGLOBIN/OXYGEN STATUS
  tHb ↓ 11.2      g/dL
  SO2     97      %
  Hct(c)   34     %
  SO2(c)   99     %
  AaDO2    0.0    mmHg
  O2Ct    15.6    vol%
  P50(c)  33.7    mmHg

ENTERED PARAMETERS
  Temp  37.0      °C
  Sex Female
  Hb Type Adult
  MCHC  3..3      %
  FIO2  0.21
  RQ    0.84
  P50   26.7      mmHg
```

- PH—7.33
- PCO_2—127
- PO_2—122
- HCO_3—65
- Na—142
- K—2.6

Interpretation: Chronic respiratory acidosis and hypokalemia—↓PH, ↑↑PCO_2, ↑↑HCO_3

ARTERIAL BLOOD GAS 7

```
le ....................................

              Results : Gass +        Normal Rage
  pH ...................... 7.123 ...... (7.3 – 7.4)
 ₂ pCO₂ ................... 64.5 ....... (35 – 48) mmHg.
   pO₂ .................... 65.1 ....... (85 – 105) mmHg.
 ₃ HCO₃ ................... 21.1 ....... (22 – 28) mmol/L.
  ecf) .................... – 8.2 ...... (-2 – +3) mmol/L.
   ...................... 83.8 % ....... (94% – 98%)

 Hct at 37⁰c.


             Results : Chem +
                                       Normal Rage
  Na⁺ ..................... 128 ........ (138 – 146) mmol/L.
  K⁺ ..................... 4.9 ........ (3.5 – 4.5) mmol/L.
  ₊ ..................... 1.02 ....... (1.15 – 1.33) mmol/L.
 ₂ ..................... 23.1 ....... (22 – 29) mmol/L.
 ⌐ ..................... 53 % ....... (% PCV)
 b ..................... 17.9 ....... (12 – 17) g/dL.
 b) ..................... – 9.7 ....... (-2 – +3) mmol/L.


             Results : META +
   ..................... 303 ........ (74 – 100) mg/dL.
   ..................... 6.52 ....... (0.56 – 1.39) mmol/L.

 PLE TYPE :– (A)
```

- PH—7.123
- PCO$_2$—64.5
- PO$_2$—65.1
- HCO$_3$—21.1
- Na—128
- K—4.9

Interpretation: Mixed acidosis—respiratory acidosis with metabolic acidosis—↓↓PH, ↑PCO$_2$, ↓HCO$_3$

ARTERIAL BLOOD GAS 8

```
ACID/BASE  37.0°C
  pH      7.44
  PCO2↓    28      mmHg
  PO2      79      mmHg
  BE       -5.1      mmol/L
  tCO2     19.3      mmol/L
  HCO3     18.4      mmol/L
  BB       39.9      mmol/L
  BEact    -4.6      mmol/L
  BEecf    -5.8      mmol/L
  stHCO3   20.3      mmol/L
  st.pH    7.329
  cH+      36.5      nmol/L

ELECTROLYTES
  Na+ ↓   113       mmol/L
  K+  ↓   3.2       mmol/L
  Ca++↓ 0.58        mmol/L
  nCa++   0.60      mmol/L

HEMOGLOBIN/OXYGEN STATUS
  tHb ↓   7.8      g/dL
  SO2 ↓   92       %
  Hct(c)    24      %
  SO2(c)    96      %
  AaDO2   38.3      mmHg
  O2Ct    10.3      vol%
  P50(c)  32.4      mmHg

ENTERED PARAMETERS
  Temp  37.0      °C
  Sex Male
  Hb Type Adult
  MCHC  33.3      %
  FIO2  0.21
  RQ   0.84
  P50  26.7      mmHg

Barometer:757.6 mmHg
Operator ID:1
S/N:9851  LOT:548402
```

- PH—7.44
- PCO_2—28
- PO_2—79
- HCO_3—18.4
- NA—113
- K—3.2

- *Interpretation*: Chronic respiratory alkalosis with severe hyponatremia and mild hypokalemia—↑PH, ↓PCO_2, ↓HCO_3
- *Causes of chronic respiratory alkalosis*:
  - Febrile condition causing hyperventilation such as pneumonia, viral infection, heart failure, etc.
  - Salicylate poisoning
  - Hysteric hyperventilation
- *Causes of hyponatremia*:
  - Hypovolemic hyponatremia
  - Euvolemic hyponatremia
  - Hypervolemic hyponatremia
- *Causes of hypokalemia*: GI loss, diuretics, metabolic alkalosis, renal loss, Conn syndrome.

ARTERIAL BLOOD GAS 9

```
Pat. ID:02
Sample No.:97

ACID/BASE  37.0°C
  pH      7.48
  PCO2↑   78       mmHg
  PO2 ↓   63       mmHg
  BE      25.7     mmol/L
  tCO2    59.4     mmol/L
  HCO3    57.0     mmol/L
  BB      75.3     mmol/L
  BEact   26.0     mmol/L
  BEecf   33.5     mmol/L
  stHCO3  47.8     mmol/L
  st.pH   7.702
  cH+     33.2     nmol/L

ELECTROLYTES
  Na+     139      mmol/L
  K+  ↓   2.3      mmol/L
  Ca++↓  1.10      mmol/L
  nCa++   1.15     mmol/L

HEMOGLOBIN/OXYGEN STATUS
  tHb ↑ 18.8       g/dL
  SO2     92       %
  Hct(c)    56     %
  SO2(c)    95     %
  AaDO2  103.2     mmHg
  O2Ct    24.3     vol%
  P50(c)  25.8     mmHg

ENTERED PARAMETERS
  Temp  37.0    °C
  Sex Male
  Hb Type Adult
  MCHC  33.3     %
  FIO2  0.36
  RQ  0.84
  P50   26.7     mmHg

Barometer:753.5 mmHg
Operator ID:
S/N:10168  LOT:348401


(Ref.Lim)
  pH     7.20  -   7.60
  PCO2    30   -    50 mmHg
  PO2     70   -   700 mmHg
  Na+    135   -   145 mmol/L
  K+      3.5  -   5.1 mmol/L
  Ca++   1.12  -  1.32 mmol/L
  tHb    12.0  -  17.0 g/dL
  SO2     90   -   100 %

MESSAGES
PCO2 over   50 (Ref.Lim)
PO2  under  70 (Ref.Lim)
K+   under 3.5 (Ref.Lim)
Ca++ under 1.12 (Ref.Lim)
tHb  over 17.0 (Ref.Lim)
```

- PH—7.48
- PCO$_2$—78
- HCO$_3$—57
- Na—139
- K—2.3
- *Interpretation*: Metabolic alkalosis due to hypokalemia with compensatory respiratory acidosis—↑PH, ↑PCO$_2$, ↑HCO$_3$

ARTERIAL BLOOD GAS 10

```
Pat. ID:002
Sample No.:289

ACID/BASE 37.0°C
 pH   ↓ 7.19
 PCO2     32      mmHg
 PO2 ↓    60      mmHg
 BE      -15.2    mmol/L
 tCO2     12.8    mmol/L
 HCO3     11.8    mmol/L
 BB       30.5    mmol/L
 BEact   -15.6    mmol/L
 BEecf   -16.4    mmol/L
 stHCO3   12.8    mmol/L
 st.pH    7.128
 cH+      64.8    nmol/L

ELECTROLYTES
 Na+ ↓   116      mmol/L
 K+  ↑   6.7      mmol/L
 Ca++↓ 1.06       mmol/L
 nCa++   0.95     mmol/L

HEMOGLOBIN/OXYGEN STATUS
 tHb ↓   9.6      g/dL
 SO2 ↓   84       %
 Hct(c)   29      %
 SO2(c)   81      %
 AaDO2   50.7     mmHg
 O2Ct    11.4     vol%
 P50(c)  32.8     mmHg

ENTERED PARAMETERS
 Temp  37.0     °C
 Sex Male
 Hb Type Adult
 MCHC   33.3     %
 FIO2   0.21
 RQ  0.84
 P50  26.7       mmHg

Barometer:745.7 mmHg
Operator ID:
S/N:10168  LOT:417400
```

- PH—7.19
- PCO_2—32
- PO_2—60
- HCO_3—11.8
- Na—116
- K—6.7

- *Interpretation*: Metabolic acidosis with severe hyponatremia and hyperkalemia probably due to renal failure—↓↓PH, ↓↓HCO_3, ↓PCO_2
- Another condition where hyponatremia with hyperkalemia is seen—Addison's disease

EXERCISE

EXERCISE 1

```
Pat. ID:01
Sample No.:1103

ACID/BASE 37.0°C
 pH   ↓ 7.07
 PCO2↑  108    mmHg
 PO2     88    mmHg
 BE      -3.1  mmol/L
 tCO2    33.7  mmol/L
 HCO3    30.4  mmol/L
 BB      44.7  mmol/L
 BEact   -4.2  mmol/L
 BEecf    0.2  mmol/L
 stHCO3  29.4  mmol/L
 st.pH  7.332
 cH+     85.6  nmol/L

ELECTROLYTES
 Na+    135    mmol/L
 K+       3.7  mmol/L
 Ca++↓  0.67   mmol/L
 nCa++   0.57  mmol/L

HEMOGLOBIN/OXYGEN STATUS
 tHb    14.7   g/dL
 SO2     93    %
 Hot(c)  44    %
 SO2(c)  91    %
 AaDO2   75.9  mmHg
 O2Ct    19.2  vol%
 P50(c) -----  mmHg

ENTERED PARAMETERS
 Temp  37.0   °C
 Sex Male
 Hb Type Adult
 MCHC  33.3   %
 FIO2  0.40
 RQ  0.84
 P50  26.7    mmHg

Barometer:758.5 mmHg
Operator ID:
S/N:9851  LOT:336401
```

- PH—7.07
- PCO_2—108
- PO_2—88
- HCO_3—30.4
- Na—135
- K—3.7

Q1. Interpret the ABG.
Q2. How to manage the patient?

EXERCISE 2

```
     Pat. ID:RCU 01
     Acc. No.:
     Sample No.:225

     ACID/BASE   37.0°C
       pH      ↓ 7.18
       PCO2    ↑    84 mmHg
       PO2     ↓    51 mmHg
       BE          -0.1 mmol/L
       LCO2        33.1 mmol/L
       HCO3        30.5 mmol/L
       BB          47.1 mmol/L
       BEact       -0.9 mmol/L
       BEecf        2.2 mmol/L
       stHCO3      23.3 mmol/L
       st.pH · 7.389
       cH+         66.2 nmol/L

     ELECTROLYTES
       Na+    ↓  130 mmol/L
       K+          4.2 mmol/L
       Ca++   ↓ 0.93 mmol/L
       nCa++     0.83 mmol/L

     HEMOGLOBIN/OXYGEN STATUS
       tHb        13.3 g/dL
       SO2    ↓    83 %
       Hct(c)      40 %
       SO2(c)      75 %
       AaDO2    425.1 mmHg
       O2Ct      15.4 vol%
       P50(c)    29.0 mmHg

     ENTERED PARAMETERS
       DOB
       Temp       37.0   °C
       Sex        Male
       Hb Type    Adult
       MCHC       33.3  %
       FIO2       0.80
       RQ         0.84
       P50        26.7   mmHg

     Barometer:751.4 mmHg
     Operator ID:
     S/N:5151   LOT:421402


     (Ref.Lim)
       pH      7.20 -   7.60
       PCO2    30 -      50 mmHg
       PO2     70 -     700 mmHg
       Na+    135 -     145 mmol/L
       K+      3.5 -     5.1 mmol/L
       Ca++   1.12 -   1.32 mmol/L
       tHb    12.0 -   17.0 g/dL
       SO2     90 -     100 %

     MESSAGES
       pH under  7.20 (Ref.Lim)
       PCO2 over   50 (Ref.Lim)
       PO2 under   70 (Ref.Lim)
       Na+ under  135 (Ref.Lim)
       Ca++ under 1.12 (Ref.Lim)
       SO2 under   90 (Ref.Lim)
       Reminder: Replace Pump
```

- PH—7.18
- PCO$_2$—84
- PO$_2$—51
- HCO$_3$—30.5
- Na—130
- K—4.2

Q1. Interpret the ABG.

Q2. What are the causes of respiratory acidosis?

EXERCISE 3

```
Pat. ID:01
Sample No.:830

ACID/BASE 37.0°C
 pH  ↓ 7.10
 PCO2↑   75      mmHg
 PO2 ↓   51      mmHg
 BE      -6.9    mmol/L
 tCO2    25.0    mmol/L
 HCO3    22.7    mmol/L
 BB      38.1    mmol/L
 BEact   -7.8    mmol/L
 BEecf   -7.0    mmol/L
 stHCO3  18.3    mmol/L
 st.pH   7.284
 cH+     79.5    nmol/L

ELECTROLYTES
 Na+  ↓  133     mmol/L
 K+      4.2     mmol/L
 Ca++↓ 0.99      mmol/L
 nCa++   0.85    mmol/L

HEMOGLOBIN/OXYGEN STATUS
 tHb ↓  7.9      g/dL
 SO2 ↓   71      %
 Hct(c)   24     %
 SO2(c)   69     %
 AaDO2  117.7    mmHg
 O2Ct    7.9     vol%
 P50(c) -----    mmHg

ENTERED PARAMETERS
 Temp  37.0     °C
 Sex Female
 Hb Type Adult
 MCHC  33.3     %
 FIO2  0.36
 RQ  0.84
 P50  26.7      mmHg

Barometer:749.8 mmHg
Operator ID:
S/N:9851  LOT:323401


(Ref.Lim)
 pH      7.20 -  7.60
 PCO2    30 -     50 mmHg
 PO2     70 -    700 mmHg
 Na+     135 -   145 mmol/L
 K+      3.5 -   5.1 mmol/L
 Ca++    1.12 -  1.32 mmol/L
 tHb     12.0 -  17.0 g/dL
 SO2     90 -    100 %

MESSAGES
 pH    under 7.20 (Ref.Lim)
 PCO2  over    50 (Ref.Lim)
 PO2   under   70 (Ref.Lim)
 Na+   under  135 (Ref.Lim)
 Ca++  under 1.12 (Ref.Lim)
 tHb   under 12.0 (Ref.Lim)
 SO2   under   90 (Ref.Lim)
```

- PH—7.10
- PCO_2—75
- PO_2—51
- HCO_3—22.7
- Na—133
- K—4.2

Q1. Interpret the ABG.

Q2. What are the causes of metabolic acidosis?

EXERCISE 4

```
ACID/BASE 37.0°C
 pH     7.50
 PCO2    33     mmHg
 PO2     72     mmHg
 BE       2.6   mmol/L
 tCO2    26.6   mmol/L
 HCO3    25.6   mmol/L
 BB      48.7   mmol/L
 BEact    3.3   mmol/L
 BEecf    2.4   mmol/L
 stHCO3  26.6   mmol/L
 st.pH  7.446
 cH+     31.5   nmol/L

ELECTROLYTES
 Na+ ↓  130     mmol/L
 K+  ↓  2.8     mmol/L
 Ca++↓ 1.00     mmol/L
 nCa++  1.05    mmol/L

HEMOGLOBIN/OXYGEN STATUS
 tHb ↓ 10.5     g/dL
 SO2     95     %
 Hct(c)   31    %
 SO2(c)   96    %
 AaDO2  114.1   mmHg
 O2Ct    14.1   vol%
 P50(c)  25.5   mmHg

ENTERED PARAMETERS
 Temp  37.0     °C
 Sex Male
 Hb Type Adult
 MCHC  33.3     %
 FIO2  0.32
 RQ    0.84
 P50   26.7     mmHg

Barometer:747.0 mmHg
Operator ID:17
S/N:9851  LOT:516402


(Ref.Lim)
 pH      7.20 -  7.60
 PCO2     30 -   50 mmHg
 PO2      70 -  700 mmHg
 Na+     135 -  145 mmol/L
 K+      3.5 -  5.1 mmol/L
 Ca++   1.12 - 1.32 mmol/L
 tHb    12.0 - 17.0 g/dL
 SO2      90 -  100 %

MESSAGES
Na+  under  135 (Ref.Lim)
K+   under  3.5 (Ref.Lim)
Ca++ under 1.12 (Ref.Lim)
tHb  under 12.0 (Ref.Lim)
```

- PH—7.50
- PCO$_2$—33
- PO$_2$—72
- HCO$_3$—25.6
- Na—130
- K—2.8

Q1. Interpret the ABG.

Q2. What are the causes of respiratory alkalosis?

EXERCISE 5

```
ACID/BASE  37.0°C
 pH   ↓ 6.98
 PCO2↑   130      mmHg
 PO2      117      mmHg
 BE       -5.2     mmol/L
 tCO2     34.2     mmol/L
 HCO3     30.2     mmol/L
 BB       32.6     mmol/L
 BEact    -6.5     mmol/L
 BEecf    -1.4     mmol/L
 stHCO3   16.5     mmol/L
 st.pH    7.290
 cH+      104.2    nmol/L

ELECTROLYTES
 Na+      137      mmol/L
 K+       4.5      mmol/L
 Ca++     1.17     mmol/L
 nCa++    0.95     mmol/L

HEMOGLOBIN/OXYGEN STATUS
 tHb      14.6     g/dL
 SO2      96       %
 Hct(c)   44       %
 SO2(c)   94       %
 AaDO2    0.0      mmHg
 O2Ct     19.9     vol%
 P50(c)   -----    mmHg

ENTERED PARAMETERS
 Temp  37.0      °C
 Sex Female
 Hb Type Adult
 MCHC  33.3      %
 FIO2  0.28
 RQ  0.84
 P50  26.7      mmHg

Barometer:747.5 mmHg
Operator ID:
S/N:9851  LOT:716401


 (Ref.Lim)
 pH      7.20 -   7.60
 PCO2    30 -     50 mmHg
 PO2     70 -     700 mmHg
 Na+     135 -    145 mmol/L
 K+      3.5 -    5.1 mmol/L
 Ca++    1.12 -   1.32 mmol/L
 tHb     12.0 -   17.0 g/dL
 SO2     90 -     100 %

MESSAGES
 pH    under 7.20 (Ref.Lim)
 PCO2  over   50 (Ref.Lim)
```

- PH—6.98
- PCO_2—130
- PO_2—117
- HCO_3—30.2
- Na—137
- K—4.5

Q1. Interpret the ABG.

Q2. How to manage the patient?

EXERCISE 6

```
Pat. ID:1
Sample No.:184

ACID/BASE 37.0°C
  pH        7.51
  PCO2      31      mmHg
  PO2       197     mmHg
  BE        1.4     mmol/L
  tCO2      25.0    mmol/L
  HCO3      24.0    mmol/L
  BB        47.8    mmol/L
  BEact     2.2     mmol/L
  BEecf     0.9     mmol/L
  stHCO3    25.6    mmol/L
  st.pH     7.430
  cH+       31.3    nmol/L

ELECTROLYTES
  Na+  ↓    131     mmol/L
  K+   ↓    2.0     mmol/L
  Ca++↓     0.54    mmol/L
  nCa++     0.57    mmol/L

HEMOGLOBIN/OXYGEN STATUS
  tHb  ↓    11.1    g/dL
  SO2       100     %
  Hct(c)    33      %
  SO2(c)    100     %
  AaDO2     0.0     mmHg
  O2Ct      15.9    vol%
  P50(c)    28.9    mmHg

ENTERED PARAMETERS
  Temp   37.0     °C
  Sex  Female
  Hb Type Adult
  MCHC   33.3     %
  FIO2   0.24
  RQ   0.84
  P50   26.7     mmHg

Barometer:755.9 mmHg
Operator ID:
S/N:9851   LOT:434401

(Ref.Lim)
  pH       7.20  -  7.60
  PCO2     30    -  50  mmHg
  PO2      70    -  100 mmHg
  Na+      135   -  145 mmol/L
  K+       3.5   -  5.1 mmol/L
  Ca++     1.12  -  1.32 mmol/L
  tHb      12.0  -  17.0 g/dL
  SO2      90    -  100 %

MESSAGES
  Na+  under  135 (Ref.Lim)
  K+   under  3.5 (Ref.Lim)
  Ca++ under  1.12 (Ref.Lim)
  Hb   under  12.0 (Ref.Lim)
```

- PH—7.51
- PCO$_2$—31
- PO$_2$—197
- HCO$_3$—24
- Na—131
- K—2.0

Q1. Interpret the ABG.

Q2. What are the causes of metabolic alkalosis?

EXERCISE 7

```
Pat. ID:17
Sample No.:357

ACID/BASE 37.0°C
 pH  ↓ 6.95
 PCO2↑  133      mmHg
 PO2    137      mmHg
 BE     -5.0     mmol/L
 tCO2   32.4     mmol/L
 HCO3   28.3     mmol/L
 BB     40.4     mmol/L
 BEact  -6.0     mmol/L
 BEecf  -3.9     mmol/L
 stHCO3 18.9     mmol/L
 st.pH  7.299
 cH+    113.4    nmol/L

ELECTROLYTES
 Na+ ↓  131      mmol/L
 K+     4.1      mmol/L
 Ca++↓ 1.05      mmol/L
 nCa++  0.83     mmol/L

HEMOGLOBIN/OXYGEN STATUS
 tHb ↓  8.8      g/dL
 SO2    97       %
 Hct(c)  26      %
 SO2(c)  96      %
 AaDO2   0.0     mmHg
 O2Ct   12.3     vol%
 P50(c) -----    mmHg

ENTERED PARAMETERS
 Temp  37.0     °C
 Sex Male
 Hb Type Adult
 MCHC  33.3     %
 FIO2  0.32
 RQ  0.84
 P50  26.7      mmHg

Barometer:749.1 mmHg
Operator ID:
S/N:10168  LOT:417400


 (Ref.Lim)
 pH     7.20 -  7.60
 PCO2    30 -    50 mmHg
 PO2     70 -   700 mmHg
 Na+    135 -   145 mmol/L
 K+     3.5 -   5.1 mmol/L
 Ca++  1.12 -  1.32 mmol/L
 tHb   12.0 -  17.0 g/dL
 SO2     90 -   100 %

MESSAGES
 pH    under 7.20 (Ref.Lim)
 PCO2  over    50 (Ref.Lim)
 Na+   under  135 (Ref.Lim)
 Ca++  under 1.12 (Ref.Lim)
 tHb   under 12.0 (Ref.Lim)
```

- PH—6.95
- PCO_2—133
- PO_2—137
- HCO_3—28.3
- Na—131
- K—4.1

Q1. What is your diagnosis?

ANSWERS

EXERCISE 1

1. Acute respiratory acidosis—$\downarrow\downarrow$PH, $\uparrow\uparrow$PCO$_2$, $\uparrow$HCO$_3$
2. The patient needs urgent mechanical ventilation followed by treatment of the primary cause.

EXERCISE 2

1. Acute respiratory acidosis—$\downarrow\downarrow$PH, $\uparrow\uparrow$PCO$_2$, $\uparrow$HCO$_3$
2. *Causes of acute respiratory acidosis*:
    a. Pulmonary cause:
        i. T2rf in COPD
        ii. Occasionally in acute exacerbation of asthma
    b. Central cause:
        i. CVA
        ii. Trauma
        iii. Drug induced
    c. Neuromuscular:
        i. Poliomyelitis
        ii. Myasthenia gravis
        iii. Kyphoscoliosis
        iv. Myopathy
    d. Miscelleneous:
        i. Obesity
        ii. Hypoventilation

EXERCISE 3

1. Mixed acidosis—$\downarrow\downarrow$PH, $\uparrow$PCO$_2$, $\downarrow$HCO$_3$
2. *Causes of metabolic acidosis*:
    a. Diabetic ketoacidosis
    b. Lactic acidosis
    c. Renal failure
    d. Ethanol poisoning
    e. GI bicarbonate loss

EXERCISE 4

1. Respiratory alkalosis with hypokalemic metabolic alkalosis—$\uparrow$PH, $\downarrow$PCO$_2$, $\uparrow$HCO$_3$
2. *Causes of respiratory alkalosis*:
    a. Febrile condition causing hyperventilation such as pneumonia, viral infection, heart failure, etc.
    b. Salicylate poisoning
    c. Hysteric hyperventilation

EXERCISE 5

1. Acute respiratory acidosis—$\downarrow\downarrow$PH, $\uparrow\uparrow$PCO$_2$, $\uparrow$HCO$_3$
2. Patient needs urgent mechanical ventilation.

EXERCISE 6

1. Metabolic alkalosis probably due to hypokalemia with respiratory alkalosis.
2. *Causes of metabolic alkalosis*:
   a. Diarrhea
   b. Vomiting
   c. Drugs—diuretic, steroid
   d. Exogenous bicarbonate load
   e. Primary aldosteronism
   f. Hypokalemia

EXERCISE 7

1. Acute respiratory acidosis—oxygen supplementation is high.

Lung Function Test

Susmita Kundu, Arya Chaudhuri

INTRODUCTION

Spirometry is a method of estimation of dynamic pulmonary functions. Basically, it measures flow of air into and from the lungs during inspiration and expiration. It is a tool for measuring the different inspiratory and expiratory lung volumes and flow.

It is by far the most common, most useful, and most convenient pulmonary function test **(Fig. 1).**

PHYSIOLOGICAL BASIS OF SPIROMETRY

Spirometry basically deals with various lung volumes and capacities. The lung volumes and capacities are as follows:

- *Tidal volume (Tv):* Amount of air that enters or leaves the lung during normal quiet respiration. Tv is around 500 mL.
- *Inspiratory reserve volume (IRV):* Amount of air that can be inspired in excess of normal Tv on maximal inspiration. It is around 3,000 mL.
- *Expiratory reserve volume (ERV):* Maximum volume of air that can be exhaled in excess of normal expiration on maximal expiration. It is around 1,100 mL.
- *Residual volume (RV):* Amount of air remaining in the lungs after maximal expiration. Normal value is around 1,200 mL.
- *Inspiratory capacity (IC):* Maximum amount of air that can be inspired in the lung after normal expiration, i.e., IC = Tv + IRV = 3,500 mL.
- *Functional residual capacity (FRC):* Volume of air that remains in the lung at the end of normal quiet expiration, i.e., FRC = ERV + RV = 2,300 mL.
- *Vital capacity (VC):* The maximum volume of air that can be exhaled from or inhaled into the lungs, i.e., VC = IRV + Tv + ERV = 4,600 mL.
- *Total lung capacity (TLC):* The volume of air that is present in the lungs after maximal inspiration, i.e., TLC = VC + RV **(Fig. 1).**

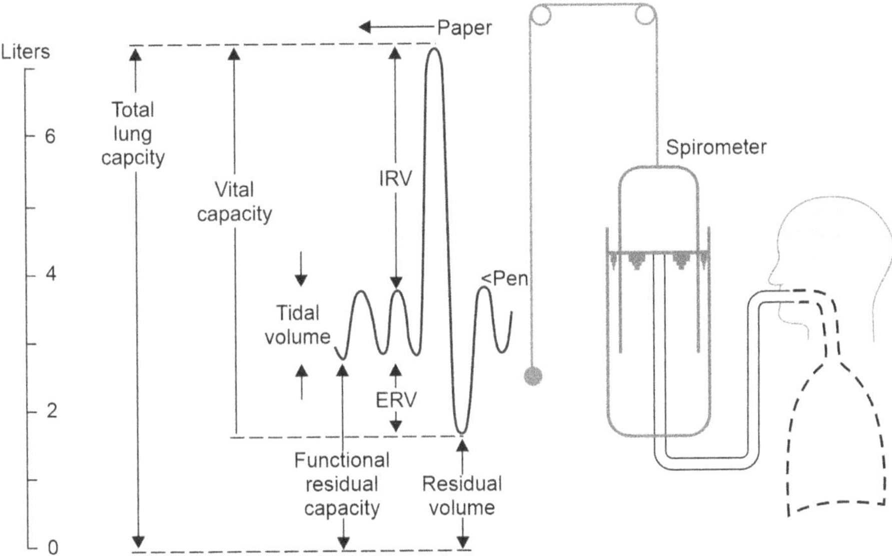

FIG. 1: The different lung volumes and capacities that can be measured by a spirometer.
(ERV: expiratory reserve volume; IRV: inspiratory reserve volume)

INDICATIONS OF SPIROMETRY

Diagnosis

- For evaluation of dynamic lung function in patients with respiratory symptoms such as cough and shortness of breath.
- Assessment of severity of different pulmonary disease (obstructive/restrictive).
- To differentiate between asthma and chronic obstructive pulmonary disease (COPD).
- To measure the physiologic effect of pulmonary disease or disorder.
- For screening of individuals at a risk of having pulmonary disease.
- Preoperative risk assessment of patients with respiratory symptoms.

Monitoring

- Assess response to therapeutic intervention.
- Monitoring of disease progression and assessment of prognosis.
- Monitoring of patients for disease exacerbation and recovery from exacerbation.
- To monitor people for adverse effects of exposure to injurious agents or drugs with known pulmonary toxicity, e.g., toxic fumes, occupational asthma, or pneumoconiosis.

Disability/Impairment Evaluation

- Assessment of patients as a part of rehabilitation program.
- Risk assessment for insurance or legal reasons.

Others

- Research and clinical trails
- Epidemiological surveys
- Pre-employment assessment for at-risk occupations.
- Health status assessment before at-risk physical activity.

RELATIVE CONTRAINDICATIONS FOR SPIROMETRY

Due to Increase in Myocardial Demand or Increased Blood Pressure

- Within 1 week of acute myocardial infarction
- Hemodynamic instability
- Significant arrhythmia
- Uncontrolled pulmonary arterial hypertension
- Severe Cor pulmonale
- Unstable pulmonary embolism
- History of cough syncope

Due to Increase in Intracranial/Intraocular Pressure

- Cerebral aneurysm
- Within 1 month of brain surgery
- Recent concussion with symptoms
- Within 1 week of eye surgery

Due to Increase in Sinus/Middle Ear Pressure

Recent sinus or middle ear surgery

Due to Increased Intrathoracic and Intra-abdominal Pressure

- Pneumothorax
- Within 1 month of thoracic or abdominal surgery
- Late-term pregnancy

Infection Control Issues

Patients with active respiratory [e.g., pulmonary tuberculosis (PTB)] or systemic infections, significant secretions or oral lesions or hemoptysis.

TYPES OF SPIROMETERS

Spirometers utilize two principles—change in volume or change in flow. Depending on that, spirometers are of two types:

1. *Volume displacement spirometers*: These record the amount of air exhaled or inhaled within a certain time.
2. *Flow sensing spirometers*: These measures how fast the air flows in or out as the volume of air inhaled or exhaled increased.

ACTIVITIES TO BE AVOIDED BEFORE PULMONARY FUNCTION TESTING

- Smoking and/or vaping 1 hour before testing.
- Consuming intoxicants within 8 hours before testing.
- Vigorous exercise within 1 hour before testing.
- Wearing tight fitting clothes that will restrict chest and abdominal expansion.

If the test is aimed at diagnosing airway disorder, then following medications should be avoided:
- Short-acting beta-2-agonist (SABA) within the last 6 hours
- Long-acting beta-2-agonist (LABA) within the last 12 hours
- Slow release theophyllines within the last 24 hours

PROCEDURE OF SPIROMETRY

- *Calibration of the spirometer*:
  - Use a 3L syringe for the same
  - The volume recorded by the spirometer during calibration should be as close as possible to 3L from the entire range of flow.
- Patient counseling and consent taking
- *Anthropometric recordings*:
  - Name
  - Age
  - Sex
  - Weight
  - Height
  - Ethnicity
    - Caucasians have the largest lung volumes.
    - Polynesians have the lowest lung volumes.
    - Approximate conversion factor for adjusting European reference values for matched Indians and 0.87 for South Indians.
- *Patient positioning*: Spirometry may be performed either in sitting or standing position.
- Defining of normal or reference values
- *Spirometric maneuver*:
  - Attach nose clips
  - Seal the lips tightly around the mouthpiece
  - Take 2–3 normal tidal breaths
  - Inhale maximally up to TLC
  - Exhale as rapidly, as forcefully, and as completely as possible (till RV)
  - Inhale rapidly till maximum capacity
  - Repeat the procedure at least three times and take the best value for interpretation

ACCEPTABILITY CRITERIA

- Back extrapolated volume (BEV) should be ≤5% of forced vital capacity (FVC) or 0.100 L, whichever is greater.
- No evidence of faulty zero-flow setting

- No cough in the 1st second of expiration
- No glottic closure after 1st second of exhalation
- No evidence of obstructed mouthpiece
- No evidence of leak
- *Must achieve one of the end of forced expiration indicators*:
  - Expiratory plateau (≤0.025 L in the last 1 second of exhalation)
  - Expiratory time ≥15 seconds
  - FVC is within repeatability tolerance of or is greater than the largest prior observed FVC.
- If the maximal inspiration after the end of forced expiration is greater than FVC, then forced inspiratory vital capacity (FIVC)-FVC must be ≤0.100 L or 5% of FVC, whichever is greater.

REPEATABILITY CRITERIA

When the age of the subject ≥6 years the difference between the two largest FVC values must be ≤0.150 L, and the difference between the two largest forced expiratory volume in 1 second (FEV1) values must be ≤0.150 L.

When the age of the subject ≤6 years (if the child is able to perform) the difference between the two largest FVC values must be ≤0.100 L or 10% of the highest value, whichever is greater.

RECORDING OF SPIROMETRY

Spirometric recording is of two types:
1. Numerical recording
2. Graphical recording

Numerical Recording of Spirometry

This refers to the various *volumes* and *flows* that can be recorded using spirometric techniques. The most important among them are:
- FEV1
- FVC
- FEV1/FVC
- Peak expiratory flow rate (PEFR)
- *Forced expiratory volume in 1 second:* This refers to the amount of air that is exhaled during the first second of the forced expiration (that is during the FVC maneuver).
- *Forced vital capacity:* The maximal volume of air forcefully exhaled after a maximal inspiration (that is inspiration up to TLC).
- *FEV1/FVC:* FEV1 in L/min divided by FVC in L/min.

Besides these values, there are some other variables that can be measured by the FVC maneuver. These values are:
- *Forced expiratory flow between 25 and 75% of vital capacity (FEF$_{25-75}$):* This refers to the FEF over middle portion of the forced expiration (that is the FVC maneuver).
- *PEF:* This is the maximal expiratory flow achieved during a maximum forced expiration initiated at TLC.
- *Peak inspiratory flow (PIF):* Maximal inspiratory flow achieved during forced inspiration to TLC.

- *Forced inspiratory flow (FIF$_{25-75}$):* Inspiratory flow over the mid portion of the forced expiratory limb.

Besides FVC, there are some other kinds of vital capacities measurable by spirometry. These vital capacities are:
- *Inspiratory vital capacity:* Starting from end-Tv the subject expires maximally and subsequently makes a full inspiration. This is the IVC.
- *Slow vital capacity (SVC):* Starting from end-Tv that subjects make a full inspiration and subsequently exhale maximally. This represents the expiratory vital capacity, or "SVC" in the Anglo-American literature.
- *Maximum voluntary ventilation (MVV):* It is the largest amount of air that a person can inhale and then exhale during a 12–15 seconds interval with maximum voluntary effort.

Volumes Not Measured by Spirometry

- *Residual volume:* Volume of air that remains in the lung after full expiration.
- *Functional residual capacity:* Amount of air that remains in the lung after normal expiration—RV + ERV.
- *Total lung capacity:* Volume of gas in the lungs after maximal inspiration—IRV + ERV + RV.

Interpretation of Spirometry (Flowchart 1)

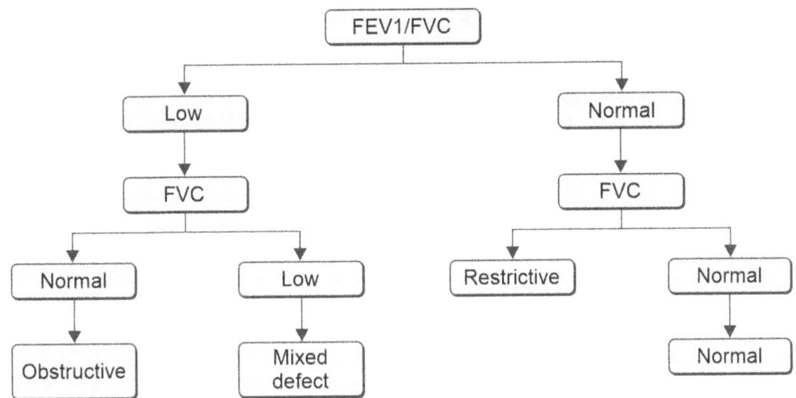

FLOWCHART 1: A flowchart for how to interpret spirometry.
(FEV1: forced expiratory volume in 1 second; FVC: forced vital capacity)

Graphical Recording of Spirometry (Fig. 2)

Graphical recording is of two types:
1. Flow volume loop
2. *Volume time curve:*
   - Volume in x axis.
   - Flow in y axis.
   - Height represents PEF.
   - Distance from TLC to 1 second mark represents FEV1 in spirometry **(Fig. 2)**.
   - Total width of the expiratory curve represents FVC.

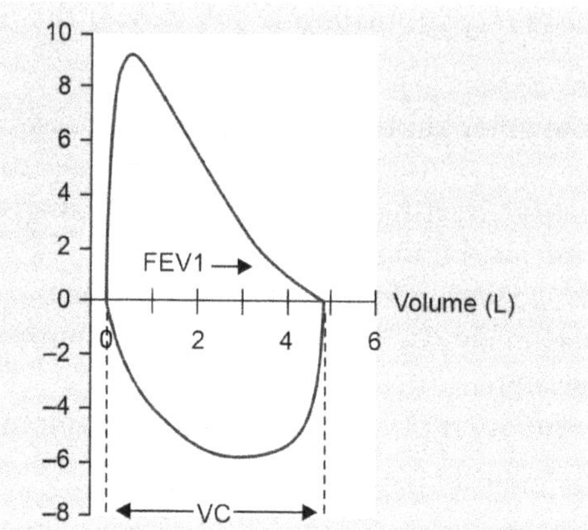

FIG. 2: Flow volume loop on a spirometry with volume on x-axis and flow on y-axis. (FEV1: forced expiratory volume in 1 second; VC: vital capacity)

Unacceptable Flow Volume Loops (Figs. 3 to 7)

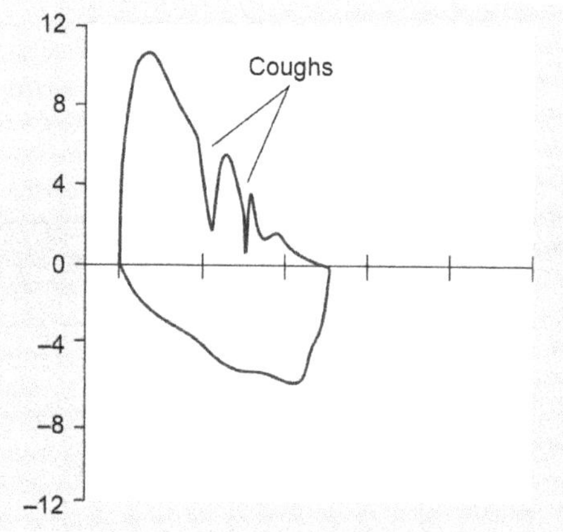

FIG. 3: Flow volume loop showing coughing during expiration while performing spirometry.

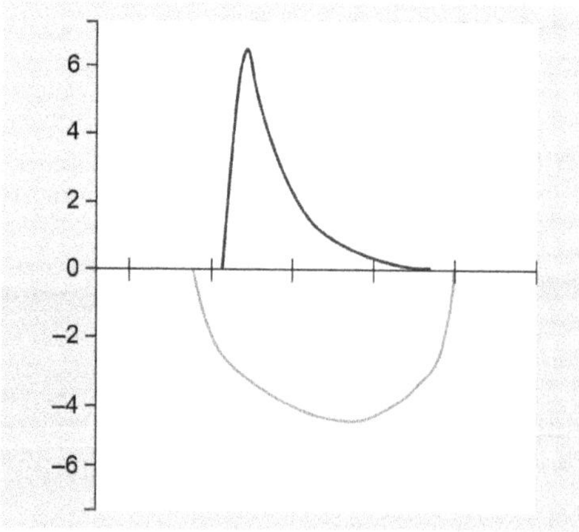

FIG. 4: Flow volume loop showing gap between expiratory flow and inspiratory flow.

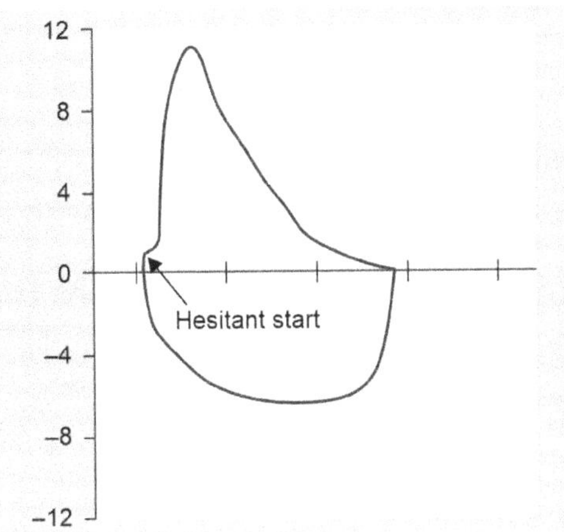

FIG. 5: Flow volume loop showing hesitant start at the beginning of expiration.

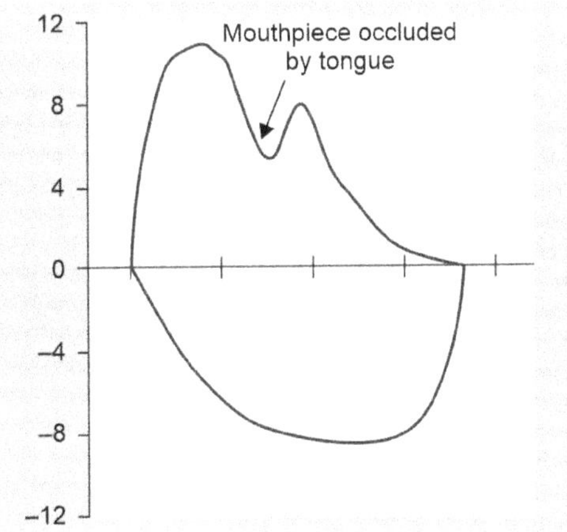

FIG. 6: Flow volume loop showing a dip in the expiratory loop due to mouthpiece occluded by tongue.

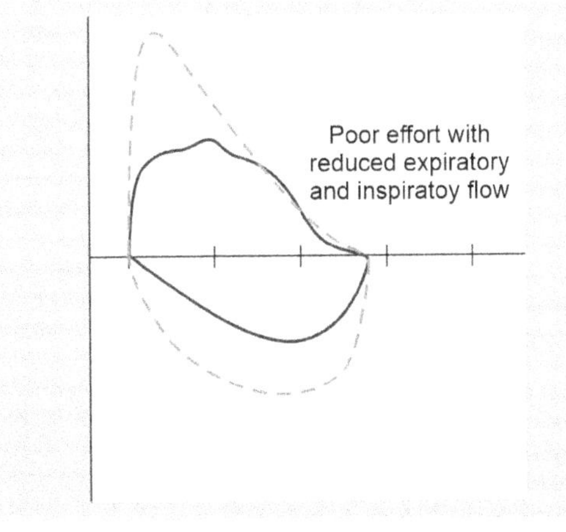

FIG. 7: Flow volume loop showing poor expiratory and inspiratory effort.

Volume Time Curve (Fig. 8)

- Time in x axis
- Volume in y axis
- FVC is represented by the highest point in the curve.
- FEV1 represented by the point in the curve that corresponds to the 1st mark **(Fig. 8)**.

Abnormalities of Flow Volume Loop in Different Diseases (Fig. 9)

Obstructive Airway Disease (Fig. 9)

Examples of obstructive airway disease are following:
- COPD
- Asthma

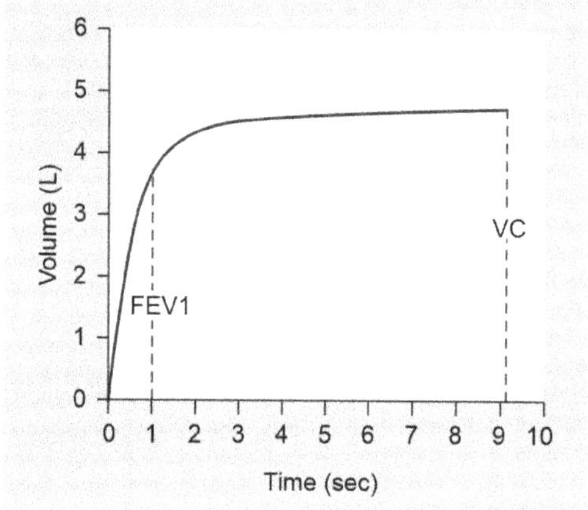

FIG. 8: A volume-time graph on spirometry.
(FEV1: forced expiratory volume in 1 second; VC: vital capacity)

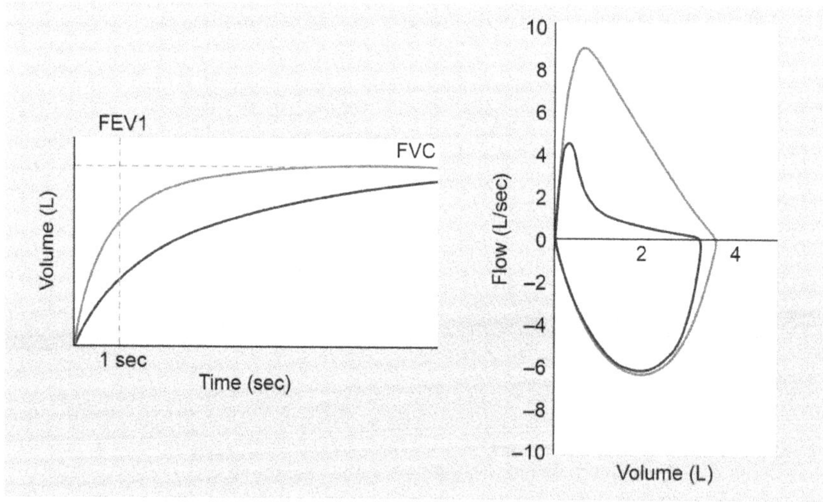

FIG. 9: Flow volume loop and volume time graph in obstructive airway disease.
(FEV1: forced expiratory volume in 1 second; FVC: forced vital capacity)

- FEV1 ↓↓
- FVC↓ or normal
- PEFR↓
- FEV1/FVC↓

Restrictive Airway Disease (Fig. 10).

Examples of restrictive airway disease are following:
- Interstitial lung disease (ILD)
- Fibrosis
- FEV1 normal or ↓
- FVC↓↓
- FEV1/FVC normal

Variable Extrathoracic Obstruction (Fig. 11)

Examples of variable extrathoracic obstruction are:
- Goiter compressing the trachea
- Hypertrophied tonsils or adenoids
- Vocal cord palsy
- Pharyngeal or laryngeal growths

Variable Intrathoracic Obstruction (Fig. 12)

Examples of variable intrathoracic obstruction are:
- Tumors of lower trachea
- Tracheomalacia
- Polychondritis of trachea
- Mediastinal mass compressing the trachea

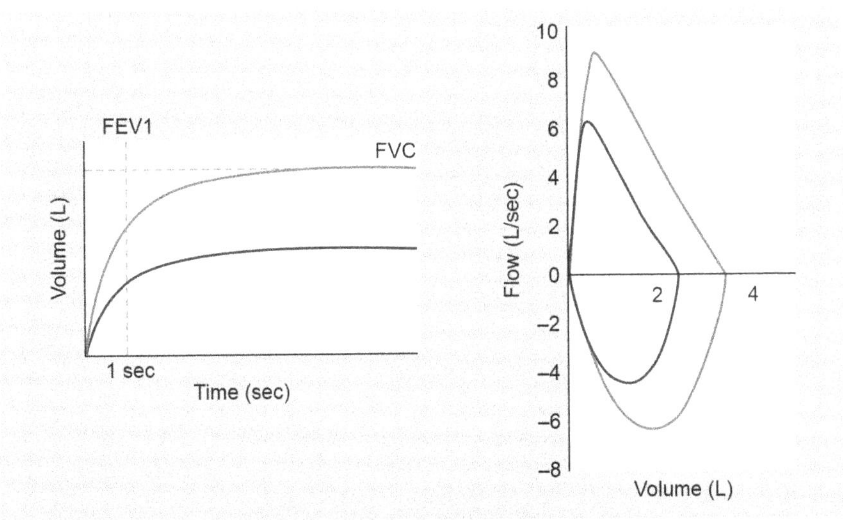

FIG. 10: Flow volume loop and volume time graph in a restrictive disease.
(FEV1: forced expiratory volume in 1 second; FVC: forced vital capacity)

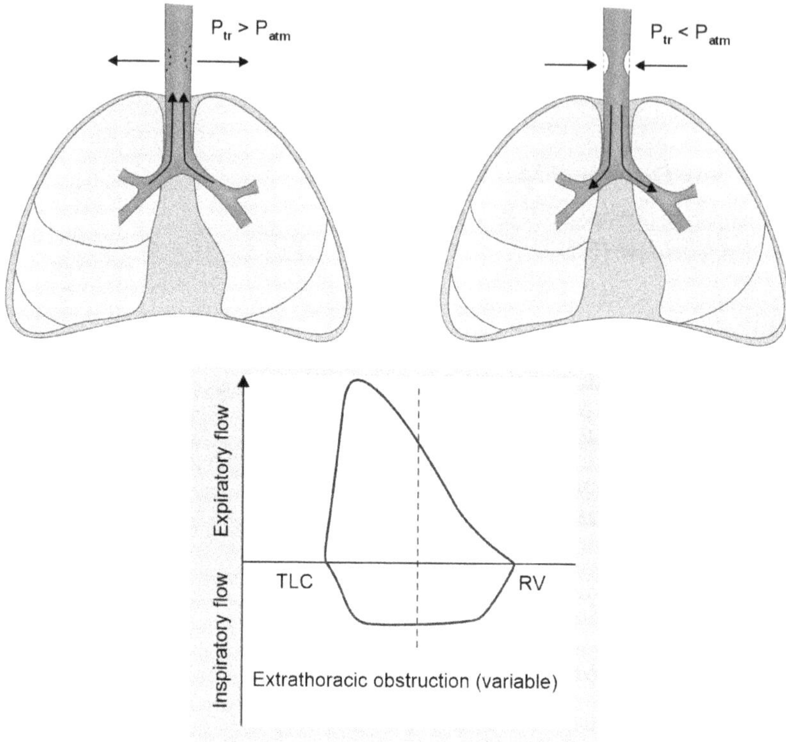

FIG. 11: Flow volume loop seen on spirometry in extrathoracic obstruction with flattening of the inspiratory limb. (TLC: Total lung capacity; RV: residual volume)

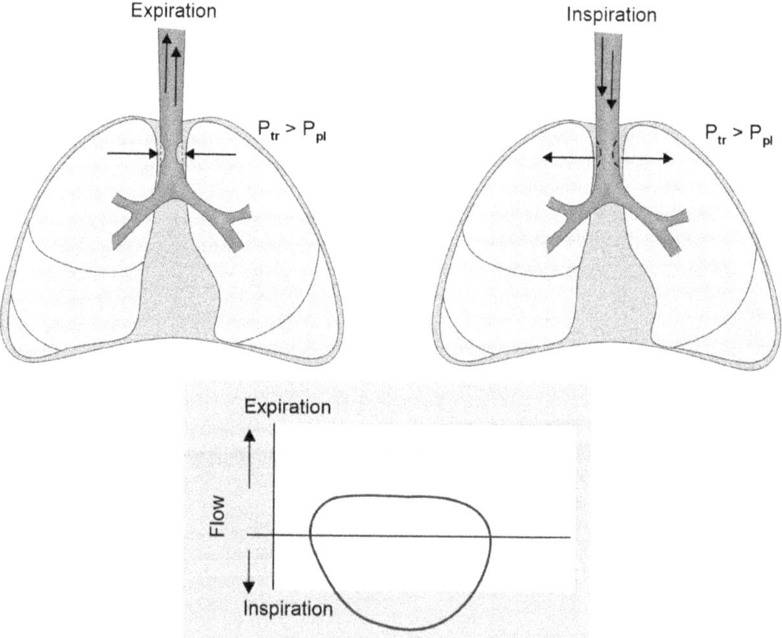

FIG. 12: Flow volume loop seen in variable intrathoracic obstruction with flattening of the expiratory curve.

Fixed Airway Obstruction (Fig. 13)

Examples of fixed airway obstruction are:
- Foreign body impaction
- Endotracheal neoplasm
- Cicatricial stenosis of trachea
- Encircling large goiter causing severe obstruction

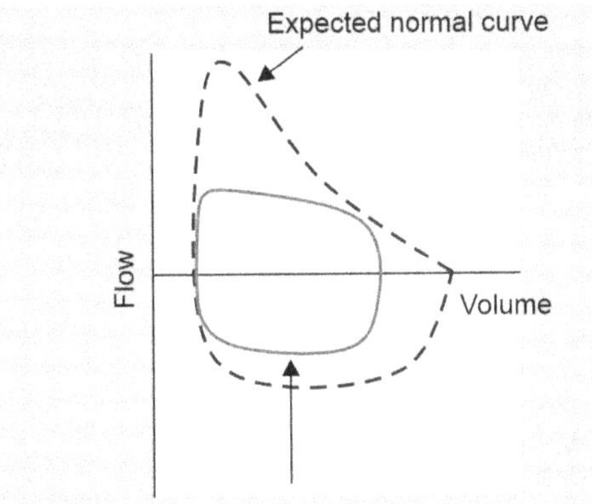

FIG. 13: Flow volume showing flattening of both the expiratory and inspiratory limb in fixed airway obstruction.

CLASSIFICATION OF CHRONIC OBSTRUCTIVE PULMONARY DISEASE ACCORDING TO SPIROMETRY (TABLE 1)

TABLE 1: Classification of COPD according to spirometry in patients with FEV1/FVC ≤ 0.7.		
Classification	**Severity**	**FEV1**
Gold 1	Mild	FEV1 ≥ 80%
Gold 2	Moderate	50% ≤ FEV1 < 80%
Gold 3	Severe	30% ≤ FEV1 < 50%
Gold 4	Very severe	FEV1 < 30%

(COPD: chronic obstructive pulmonary disease; FEV1: forced expiratory volume in 1 second; FVC: forced vital capacity)

CLASSIFICATION OF ASTHMA ACCORDING TO SPIROMETRY (TABLE 2)

TABLE 2: Classification of asthma according to spirometry.	
Severity	**FEV1**
Intermittent	≥80%
Mild persistant	≥80%
Moderate persistant	60–80%
Severe persistant	≤60%

(FEV1: forced expiratory volume in 1 second)

Spirometry 1 (Table 3)

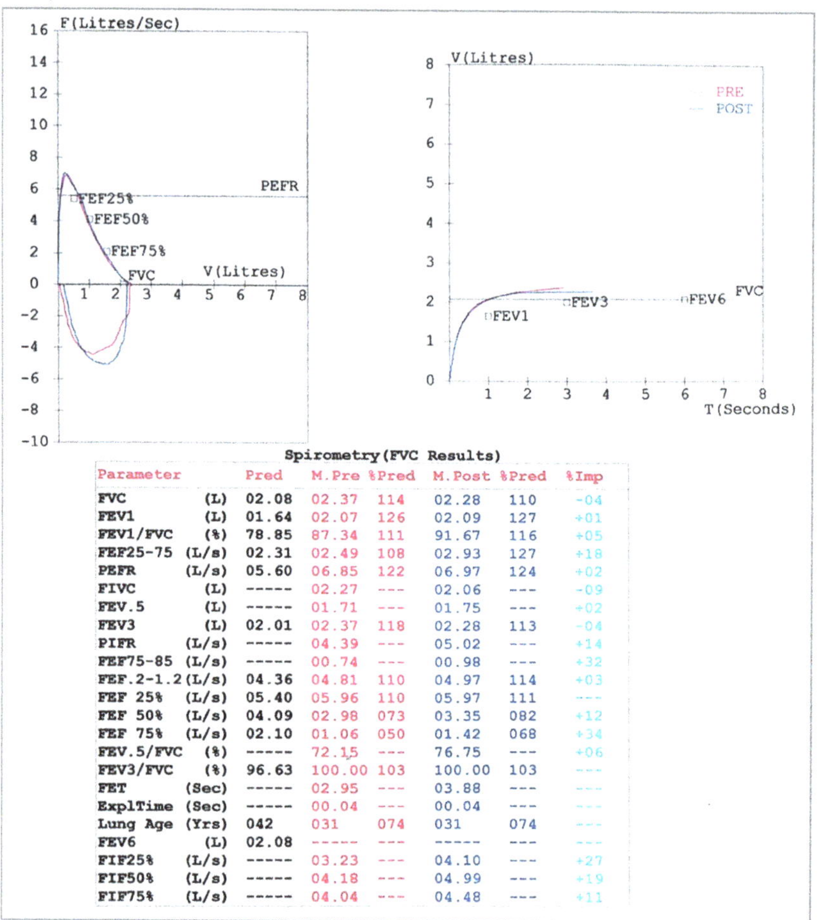

Spirometry (FVC Results)

Parameter		Pred	M.Pre	%Pred	M.Post	%Pred	%Imp
FVC	(L)	02.08	02.37	114	02.28	110	-04
FEV1	(L)	01.64	02.07	126	02.09	127	+01
FEV1/FVC	(%)	78.85	87.34	111	91.67	116	+05
FEF25-75	(L/s)	02.31	02.49	108	02.93	127	+18
PEFR	(L/s)	05.60	06.85	122	06.97	124	+02
FIVC	(L)	-----	02.27	---	02.06	---	-09
FEV.5	(L)	-----	01.71	---	01.75	---	+02
FEV3	(L)	02.01	02.37	118	02.28	113	-04
PIFR	(L/s)	-----	04.39	---	05.02	---	+14
FEF75-85	(L/s)	-----	00.74	---	00.98	---	+32
FEF.2-1.2	(L/s)	04.36	04.81	110	04.97	114	+03
FEF 25%	(L/s)	05.40	05.96	110	05.97	111	---
FEF 50%	(L/s)	04.09	02.98	073	03.35	082	+12
FEF 75%	(L/s)	02.10	01.06	050	01.42	068	+34
FEV.5/FVC	(%)	-----	72.15	---	76.75	---	+06
FEV3/FVC	(%)	96.63	100.00	103	100.00	103	---
FET	(Sec)	-----	02.95	---	03.88	---	---
ExplTime	(Sec)	-----	00.04	---	00.04	---	---
Lung Age	(Yrs)	042	031	074	031	074	---
FEV6	(L)	02.08	-----	---	-----	---	---
FIF25%	(L/s)	-----	03.23	---	04.10	---	+27
FIF50%	(L/s)	-----	04.18	---	04.99	---	+19
FIF75%	(L/s)	-----	04.04	---	04.48	---	+11

TABLE 3: Findings of spirometry 1.

Test	Predicted	Pre BDR	Post BDR	Change
FVC	02.08L	02.37	02.28	
FVC (Obs/Pred)		114%	110%	–04%
FEV1	01.64L	02.07	02.09	
FEV1 (Obs/Pred)		126%	127%	+01%
FEV1/FVC		87.34%	91.67%	
FEF$_{25-75}$	02.31L	02.49	02.93	
FEF$_{25-75}$ (Obs/Pred)		108%	127%	+18%
PEF%	05.60L	06.85	06.97	

(BDR: bronchodilator; FEV1: forced expiratory volume in 1 second; FVC: forced vital capacity; PEF: peak expiratory flow)

- *Interpretation:* This patient's FEV1, FVC, FEV1/FVC, and PEF are within normal limit. Postbronchodilator FEV1, PEF have insignificant improvement.
- This is a normal spirometry.

Spirometry 2 (Table 4)

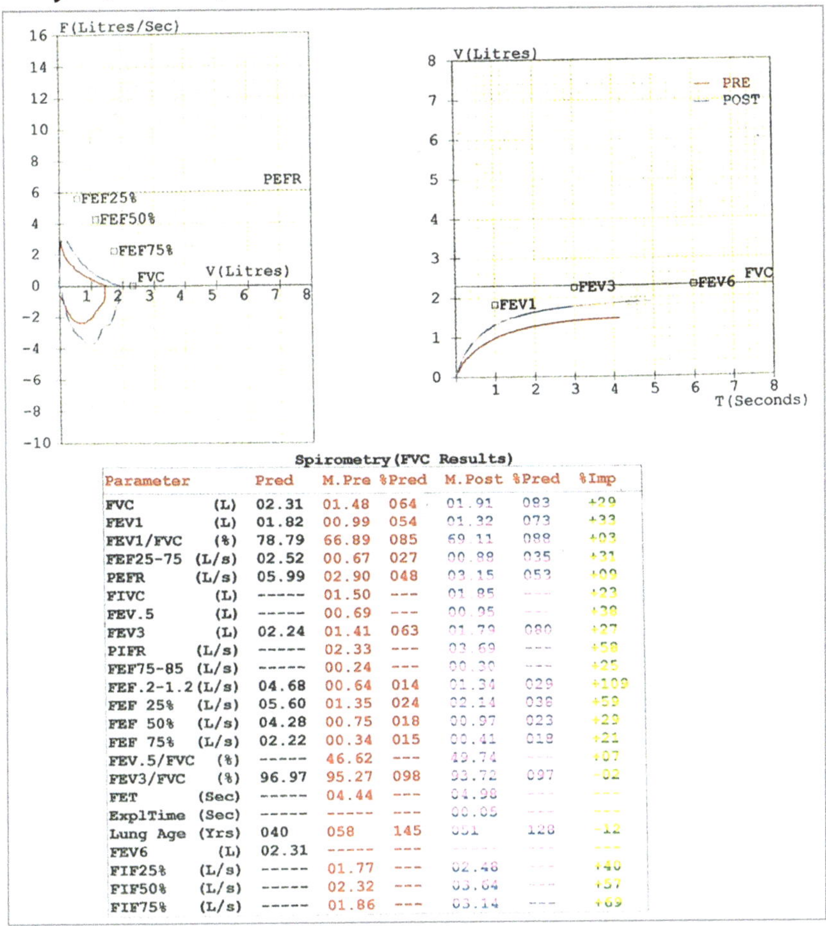

Spirometry (FVC Results)

Parameter		Pred	M.Pre	%Pred	M.Post	%Pred	%Imp
FVC	(L)	02.31	01.48	064	01.91	083	+29
FEV1	(L)	01.82	00.99	054	01.32	073	+33
FEV1/FVC	(%)	78.79	66.89	085	69.11	088	+03
FEF25-75	(L/s)	02.52	00.67	027	00.88	035	+31
PEFR	(L/s)	05.99	02.90	048	03.15	053	+09
FIVC	(L)	------	01.50	---	01.85	---	+23
FEV.5	(L)	------	00.69	---	00.95	---	+38
FEV3	(L)	02.24	01.41	063	01.79	080	+27
PIFR	(L/s)	------	02.33	---	03.69	---	+58
FEF75-85	(L/s)	------	00.24	---	00.30	---	+25
FEF.2-1.2	(L/s)	04.68	00.64	014	01.34	029	+109
FEF 25%	(L/s)	05.60	01.35	024	02.14	038	+59
FEF 50%	(L/s)	04.28	00.75	018	00.97	023	+29
FEF 75%	(L/s)	02.22	00.34	015	00.41	018	+21
FEV.5/FVC	(%)	------	46.62	---	49.74	---	+07
FEV3/FVC	(%)	96.97	95.27	098	93.72	097	-02
FET	(Sec)	------	04.44	---	04.98	---	---
ExplTime	(Sec)	------	------	---	00.05	---	---
Lung Age	(Yrs)	040	058	145	051	128	-12
FEV6	(L)	02.31	------	---			---
FIF25%	(L/s)	------	01.77	---	02.48	---	+40
FIF50%	(L/s)	------	02.32	---	03.64	---	+57
FIF75%	(L/s)	------	01.86	---	03.14	---	+69

TABLE 4: Findings of spirometry 2.

Test	Predicted	Pre BDR	Post BDR	Change
FVC	02.31L	01.48	01.91	
FVC (Obs/Pred)		64	83	+29%
FEV1	01.82L	00.99	01.32	330 mL
FEV1 (Obs/Pred)		54%	73%	+33%
FEV1/FVC		85%	88%	
FEF$_{25-75}$	02.52L	00.67	00.88	
FEF$_{25-75}$ (Obs/Pred)		27%	35%	
PEF%	05.99L	02.90	03.15	9%

(BDR: bronchodilator; FEV1: forced expiratory volume in 1 second; FVC: forced vital capacity; PEF: peak expiratory flow)

- *Interpretation:* In this patient FEV1/FVC ratio is within normal limit. There is significant improvement in postbronchodilator FEV1 (33% and 330 mL). As per GINA guideline 2023, increase in FEV1 of >12% and 200 mL (greater confidence if FEV1 increases by >15% and 400 mL) is suggestive of reversible obstructive lung disease—asthma.

- This patient has FEV1/FVC ratio >0.70. Probably this patient is having air-trapping causing significant reduction in FVC and false normalization of FEV1/FVC.

Spirometry 3 (Table 5)

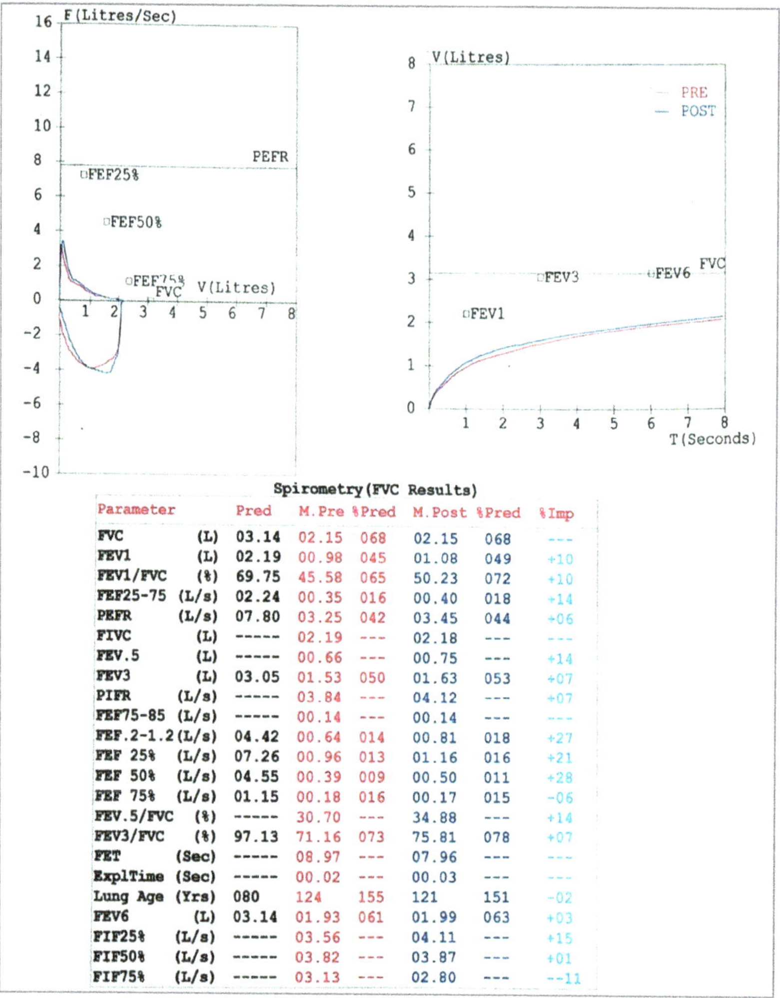

Spirometry (FVC Results)

Parameter		Pred	M.Pre	%Pred	M.Post	%Pred	%Imp
FVC	(L)	03.14	02.15	068	02.15	068	---
FEV1	(L)	02.19	00.98	045	01.08	049	+10
FEV1/FVC	(%)	69.75	45.58	065	50.23	072	+10
FEF25-75	(L/s)	02.24	00.35	016	00.40	018	+14
PEFR	(L/s)	07.80	03.25	042	03.45	044	+06
FIVC	(L)	------	02.19	---	02.18	---	---
FEV.5	(L)	------	00.66	---	00.75	---	+14
FEV3	(L)	03.05	01.53	050	01.63	053	+07
PIFR	(L/s)	------	03.84	---	04.12	---	+07
FEF75-85	(L/s)	------	00.14	---	00.14	---	---
FEF.2-1.2	(L/s)	04.42	00.64	014	00.81	018	+27
FEF 25%	(L/s)	07.26	00.96	013	01.16	016	+21
FEF 50%	(L/s)	04.55	00.39	009	00.50	011	+28
FEF 75%	(L/s)	01.15	00.18	016	00.17	015	-06
FEV.5/FVC	(%)	------	30.70	---	34.88	---	+14
FEV3/FVC	(%)	97.13	71.16	073	75.81	078	+07
FET	(Sec)	------	08.97	---	07.96	---	---
ExplTime	(Sec)	------	00.02	---	00.03	---	---
Lung Age	(Yrs)	080	124	155	121	151	-02
FEV6	(L)	03.14	01.93	061	01.99	063	+03
FIF25%	(L/s)	------	03.56	---	04.11	---	+15
FIF50%	(L/s)	------	03.82	---	03.87	---	+01
FIF75%	(L/s)	------	03.13	---	02.80	---	--11

TABLE 5: Findings of spirometry 3.				
Test	**Predicted**	**Pre BDR**	**Post BDR**	**Change**
FVC	03.14L	02.15	02.15	
FVC (Obs/Pred)		68%	68%	10%
FEV1	02.19L	00.98	01.08	
FEV1 (Obs/Pred)		45%	49%	10%
FEV1/FVC		65%	72%	
FEF$_{25-75}$	02.24L	00.35L	00.40L	
FEF$_{25-75}$ (Obs/Pred)		16%	18%	
PEF%	07.80L	00.35	00.40	6%

(BDR: bronchodilator; FEV1: forced expiratory volume in 1 second; FVC: forced vital capacity; PEF: peak expiratory flow)

- *Interpretation*: In this patient post-BDR FEV1/FVC is 0.72. But this patient is having post-BDR FEV1 49%, suggestive of moderate airway obstruction without significant bronchodilator reversibility. So, this is a case of COPD but as per 2024 Gold guideline it may fulfil criteria for PRISM (preserved ratio with impaired spirometry) as post-BDR FEV1/FVC >0.70.

Spirometry 4 (Table 6)

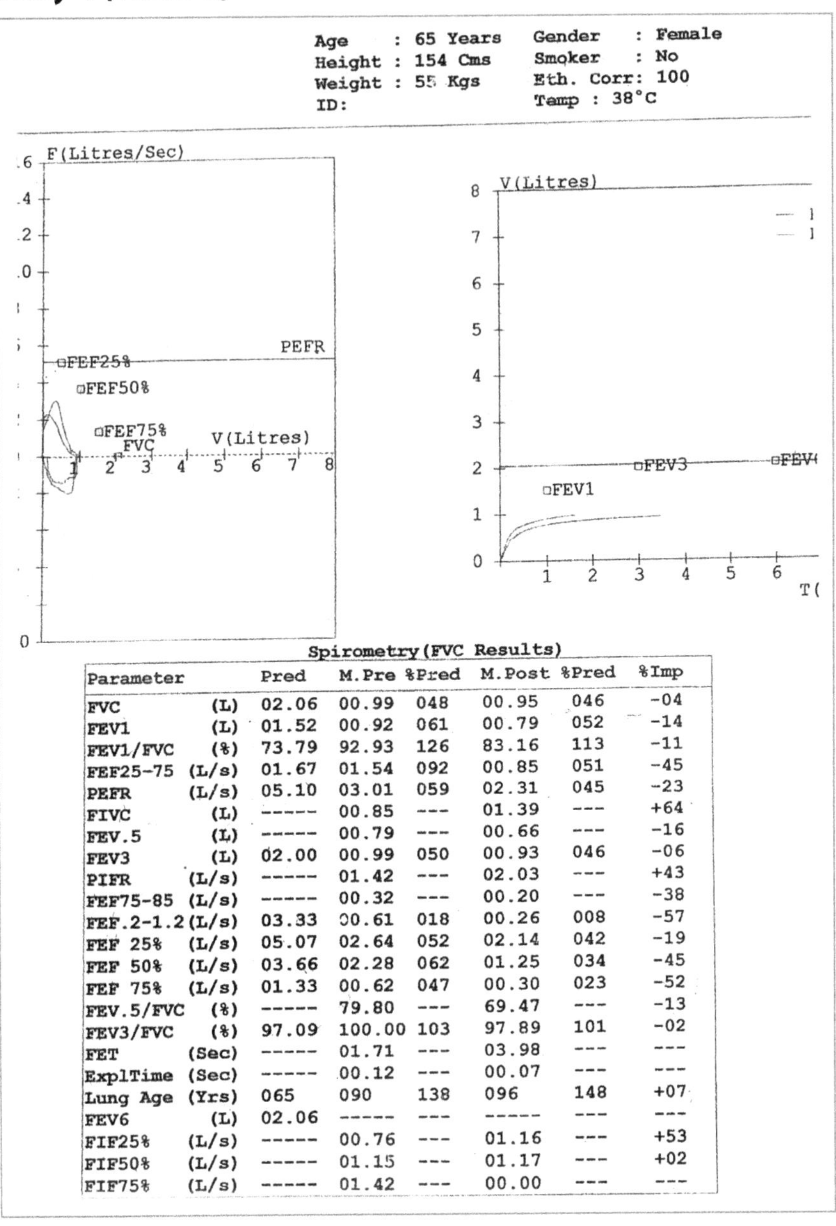

Spirometry (FVC Results)

Parameter		Pred	M.Pre	%Pred	M.Post	%Pred	%Imp
FVC	(L)	02.06	00.99	048	00.95	046	−04
FEV1	(L)	01.52	00.92	061	00.79	052	−14
FEV1/FVC	(%)	73.79	92.93	126	83.16	113	−11
FEF25−75	(L/s)	01.67	01.54	092	00.85	051	−45
PEFR	(L/s)	05.10	03.01	059	02.31	045	−23
FIVC	(L)	−−−−−	00.85	−−−	01.39	−−−	+64
FEV.5	(L)	−−−−−	00.79	−−−	00.66	−−−	−16
FEV3	(L)	02.00	00.99	050	00.93	046	−06
PIFR	(L/s)	−−−−−	01.42	−−−	02.03	−−−	+43
FEF75−85	(L/s)	−−−−−	00.32	−−−	00.20	−−−	−38
FEF.2−1.2	(L/s)	03.33	00.61	018	00.26	008	−57
FEF 25%	(L/s)	05.07	02.64	052	02.14	042	−19
FEF 50%	(L/s)	03.66	02.28	062	01.25	034	−45
FEF 75%	(L/s)	01.33	00.62	047	00.30	023	−52
FEV.5/FVC	(%)	−−−−−	79.80	−−−	69.47	−−−	−13
FEV3/FVC	(%)	97.09	100.00	103	97.89	101	−02
FET	(Sec)	−−−−−	01.71	−−−	03.98	−−−	−−−
ExplTime	(Sec)	−−−−−	00.12	−−−	00.07	−−−	−−−
Lung Age	(Yrs)	065	090	138	096	148	+07
FEV6	(L)	02.06	−−−−−	−−−	−−−−−	−−−	−−−
FIF25%	(L/s)	−−−−−	00.76	−−−	01.16	−−−	+53
FIF50%	(L/s)	−−−−−	01.15	−−−	01.17	−−−	+02
FIF75%	(L/s)	−−−−−	01.42	−−−	00.00	−−−	−−−

TABLE 6: Findings of spirometry 4.

Test	Predicted	Pre BDR	Post BDR	Change
FVC	02.06L	00.99	00.95	
FVC (Obs/Pred)		48%	46%	–04%
FEV1	01.52L	00.92	00.79	
FEV1 (Obs/Pred)		61	52%	–14%
FEV1/FVC		126%	113%	
FEF_{25-75}	01.67L	01.54L	00.85	
FEF_{25-75} (Obs/Pred)		92%	51%	
PEF%	05.10L	03.01	02.31	–23%

(BDR: bronchodilator; FEV1: forced expiratory volume in 1 second; FVC: forced vital capacity; PEF: peak expiratory flow)

- *Interpretation:* In this patient FEV1/FVC ratio is increased with a parallel decrease in FVC and FEV1, which is suggestive of restrictive ventilator defect.

CARE OF SPIROMETER

- Maximum chances of infection are with MVV and inspiratory maneuvers. Therefore, clean the tubing and the mouthpiece of the spirometer before and after doing these tests.
- Tubing of spirometer should be cleaned daily by immersing it in disinfectant solution.
- Use disposable cardboard mouthpieces.

PEAK FLOW METER TESTING

The peak flow meter is a device, which records PEFR, which correlates with FEV1 in measurements of air-flow obstruction and carrying out reversibility tests.

The air flow which enters the flow meter causes displacement of the diaphragm thereby compressing or stretching the spring or the metal plate. This displacement is proportional to the peak flow and a calibrated scale is printed on it.

"Personal best PEFR" is a better index for self-monitoring. Useful clinical indices are: Reduction in PEFR, PEFR variability, PEFR reversibility, and PEFR/PIF ratio. The difference of the highest and the lowest PEFR expressed as percent of the lowest value is termed as diurnal PEFR variability. Severity of asthma is proportional to reduction in PEFR and increase in PEFR variability. More than 20% PEFR reversibility or variability is diagnostic of asthma. Diurnal variability in PEFR is an excellent index which correlates closely with airway hyperresponsiveness. Steroid reversibility is done when the patient is suspected of having asthma but bronchodilator reversibility test is nonconfirmatory. A trial of glucocorticoids (30 mg prednisolone daily for 2 weeks) may be useful in establishing the diagnosis of asthma, by demonstrating an improvement in either FEV1 or PEF in comparison with baseline values.

Uses of Peak Flow Meter

1. To measure the PEFR for diagnosis of variable expiratory air flow in asthma.
2. Self-monitoring of asthma patients at home as a part of self-asthma management plan. For self-monitoring "personal best PEFR" is a better index.
3. Diagnosis and management of occupational asthma **(Figs. 14 and 15)**.

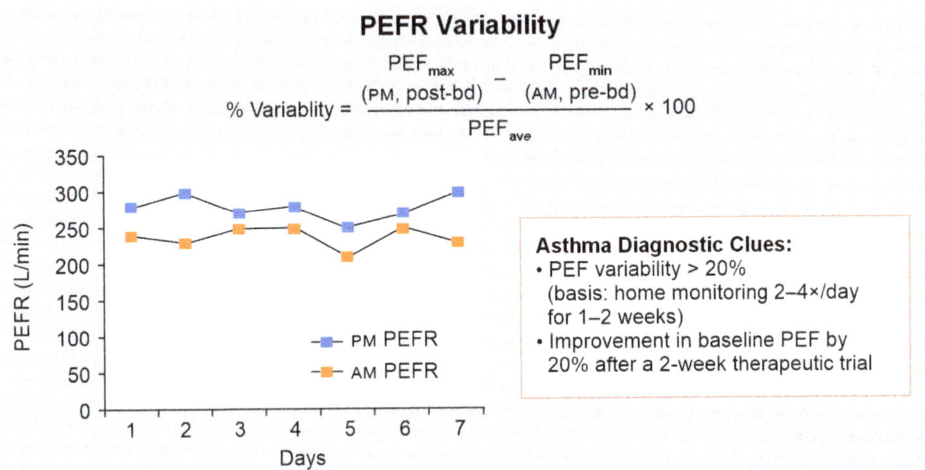

FIG. 14: Graph showing PEFR variability.

(BD: bronchodilator; PEFR: peak expiratory flow rate)

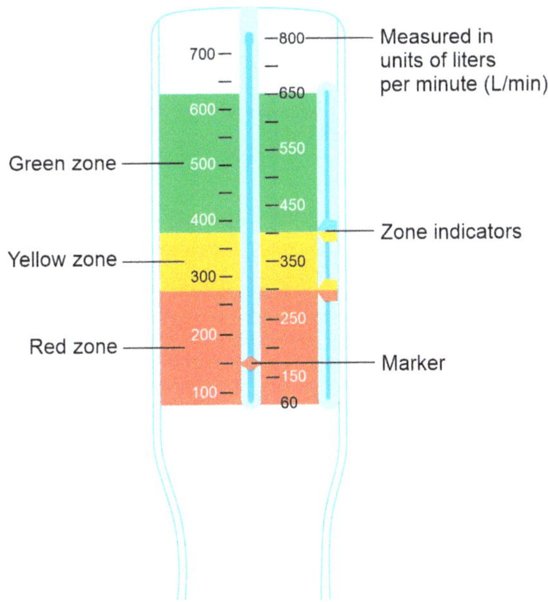

FIG. 15: Picture of a peak flow meter.

Peak Expiratory Flow Rate Zone Monitoring (Table 7)

TABLE 7: Peak expiratory flow rate zone monitoring.		
Green zone	**80–100% of usual or normal peak flow readings**	**Indicates asthma is under good control**
Yellow zone	50–79% of usual or normal peak flow readings	Indicates caution. Airways are narrowing and additional medications required or just increasing the dose of medications may suffice
Red zone	<50% of usual or normal peak flow readings	Indicates medical emergency. Severe airway narrowing and immediate action required which involves contacting a doctor or hospital

▣ DIFFUSING CAPACITY FOR CARBON MONOXIDE

The DLCO stands for diffusion capacity of lungs for carbon monoxide. It measures the ability of the lung to transfer gas from inhaled air to the red blood cells (RBCs) in pulmonary circulation. It is also known as transfer factor. It depends on the solubility, weight, and diffusion ability of gas and the thickness of the barrier (thicker barrier—decreased diffusion).

Oxygen passes through the blood gas barrier, enters RBC, and binds with hemoglobin (Hb). Blood gas barrier consists of alveolar epithelium, basement membrane, interstitium, and capillary endothelium. Abnormality in any component will affect the diffusion of oxygen (O_2).

It obeys Fick's law of diffusion:
- $V_{gas} = A \times D/T \ (P1\text{-}P2)$
- V_{gas} = Volume of gas diffusing the tissue barrier per unit time
- A = Surface area available for diffusion
- D = Diffusion coefficient
- T = Thickness of the barrier
- P1–P2 = Partial pressure difference of the gas

$$1/DLCO = 1/DM_{CO} + 1/_{CO}V_C$$
DM_{CO} = diffusing capacity of the alveolar–capillary membrane for CO
$_{CO}$ = the rate of displacement of O_2 from intracellular hemoglobin by CO
V_C = volume of blood in the pulmonary capillary bed

Importance of carbon monoxide (CO):
- High affinity for Hb (more than O_2).
- *Diffusion limited:* Less factors influence the movement of CO.
- Present in negligible amount in blood.
- Back pressure is low.

O_2 cannot be used because of the following reasons:
- Movement is influenced by ventilation
- Perfusion
- Amount of shunt
- PaO_2 (produces back pressure)

Indications for Diffusing Capacity for Carbon Monoxide

- Evaluation of dyspnea
- Early diagnosis of ILD
- Assess progression of idiopathic pulmonary fibrosis (IPF)
- Diagnosis of progressive pulmonary fibrosis (PPF)
- Evaluation of pulmonary vascular disease
- Assess drug toxicity
- Evaluation of pulmonary hemorrhage
- To diagnose and differentiate between obstructive and restrictive airway diseases.

Contraindications for Diffusing Capacity for Carbon Monoxide

Absolute Contraindications

- Presence of CO toxicity
- Severe O_2 desaturation without O_2 supplementation

Relative Contraindication

- Uncooperative patients
- Large meal or vigorous exercise immediately before the test
- Smoking within 24 hours
- Decreased lung volume that would not yield valid test results

Procedure

- Patient is asked to take 2–3 normal tidal breaths
- Patient inhales maximally
- Patients exhale to RV
- Inhales a mixture of predetermined tracer gas and CO
- Patients hold breath for 10 seconds
- CO reaches the alveolar membrane and diffuses across it. CO crosses the RBC membrane and binds with Hb.
- Subject exhales to RV
- Exhaled gas is analyzed

  Gas mixture = 0.3% CO + 0–14% helium (He) + 21% O_2 + Rest is molecular nitrogen (N2)

Preparation

- No smoking on the day of the test
- No use of bronchodilators on the day of the test
- No supplemental O_2 for at least 15 minutes prior to and during the test as O_2 supplementation can decrease DLCO by 0.35%.

Precaution

- The inspiratory volume should be greater than 85% of largest VC.
- Inspiratory time should be ideally <2 seconds.
- The sample collection time should be <3 seconds.
- The first 0.75–1 L is discarded as dead space gas. Next sample volume of 0.5–1 L is collected for analysis.

Different Methods

- Single breath holding method
- Single rebreathing method
- Intrabreath method
- Three gas iteration method
- Steady state method

$$1/DLCO = 1/D_M + 1/\varnothing V_C$$

DLCO depends on:
- D_M: Membrane diffusion
- $\varnothing$: Rate of displacement of O_2 from Hb by CO
- V_c: Alveolar capillary blood volume

Factors Affecting Diffusing Capacity for Carbon Monoxide

Factors which increase DLCO are:
- *Müller's maneuver:* Deep rapid breath against closed glottis causes increased venous return which increases the blood flow to lungs.
- Polycythemia
- High altitude
- *Supine position*: Increased venous return
- Obesity
- *Exercise*: Increased cardiac output
- Left to right shunt
- Low breath holding time
- Diffuse alveolar hemorrhage

Factors which Decreases DLCO

- Submaximal inspiration
- Valsalva maneuver
- Smoking
- Anemia
- Reduced lung volume

Correction Factor for DLCO

- DLCO (predicted for Hb) = DLCO (predicted) × (1.7 × Hb)/(10.22 + Hb)
- DLCO (predicted for altitude) = DLCO predicted/[1.0 + 0.0031 (PIO$_2$ – 150)]
- DLCO (predicted for COHb) = DLCO (predicted) × (102% – COHb%)

CO transfer coefficient (Kco):
- Transfer coefficient for the diffusion of CO into the blood (DLCO/Va)
- To correct for loss of alveolar volume
- In postlung resection—low DLCO but DLCO/Va is normal

Classification and severity of DLCO reduction:
- Normal >75% of predicted, up to 140%
- Mild decrease, 60–74%
- Moderate decrease, 40–59%
- Severe decrease, <40%

▨ CHRONOLOGICAL EVALUATION IN PULMONARY FUNCTION TEST (FLOWCHART 2)

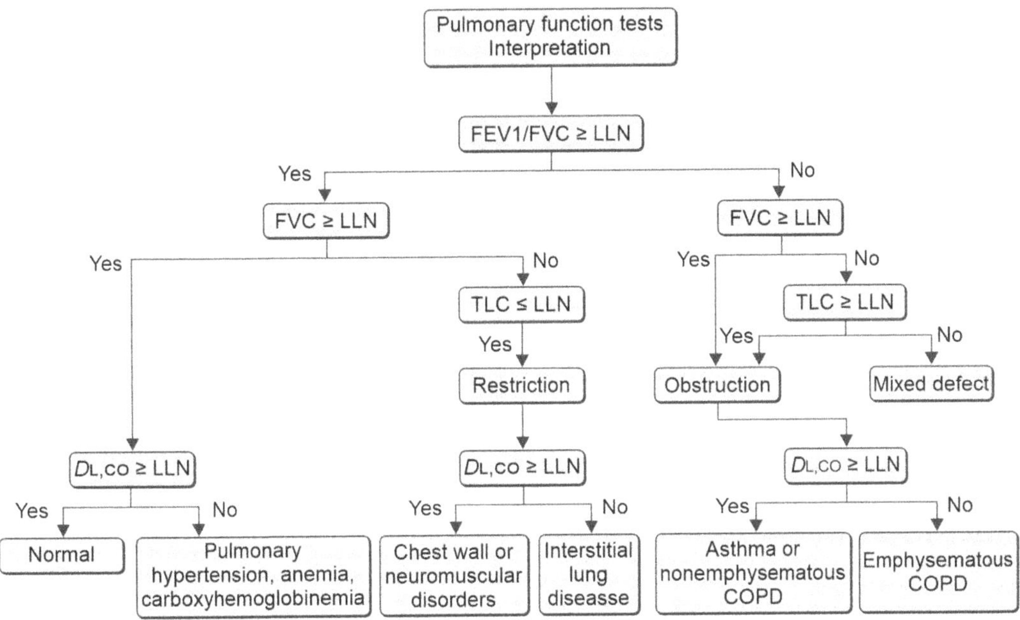

FLOWCHART 2: Algorithm for interpretation of DLCO.

(DLCO: diffusing capacity for carbon monoxide; FEV1: forced expiratory volume in 1 second; FVC: forced vital capacity; LLN: lower limit of normal; TLC: total lung capacity)

Source: Pellegrino R, Viegi G, Brusasco V, Crapo RO, Burgos F, Casaburi R, et al. Interpretative strategies for lung function tests. Eur Respir J. 2005;26(5):948-68.

◼ DIFFUSING CAPACITY FOR CARBON MONOXIDE 1

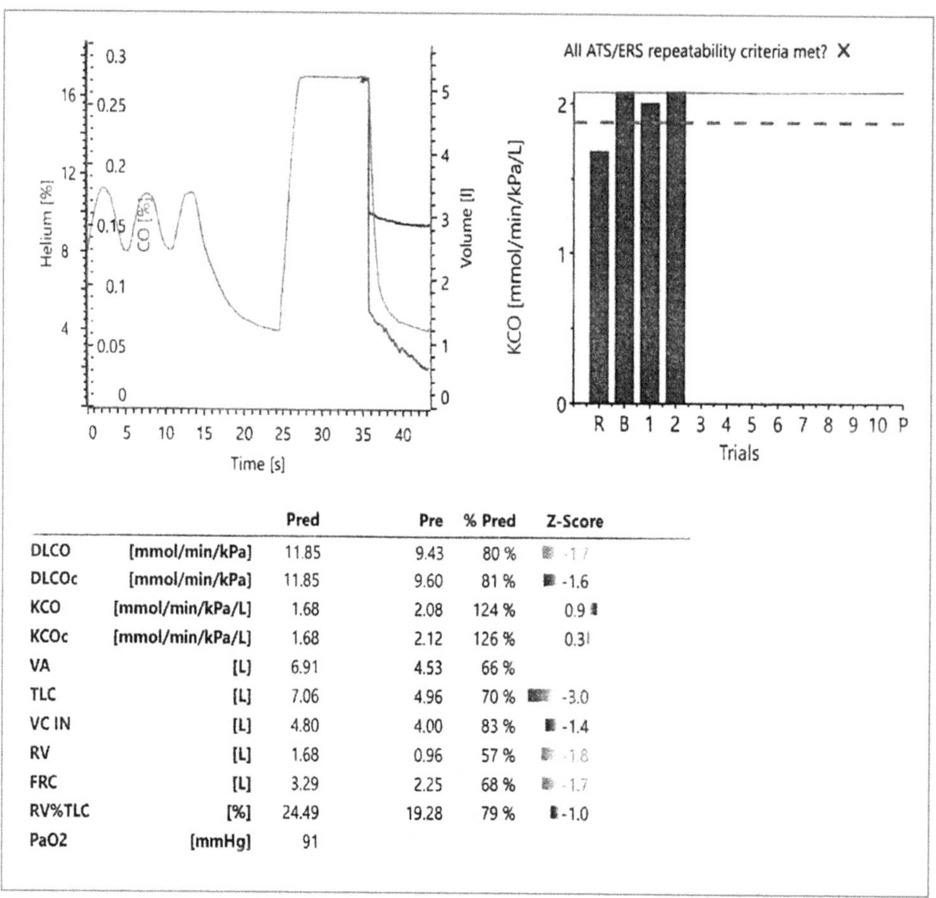

		Pred	Pre	% Pred	Z-Score
DLCO	[mmol/min/kPa]	11.85	9.43	80 %	-1.7
DLCOc	[mmol/min/kPa]	11.85	9.60	81 %	-1.6
KCO	[mmol/min/kPa/L]	1.68	2.08	124 %	0.9
KCOc	[mmol/min/kPa/L]	1.68	2.12	126 %	0.3
VA	[L]	6.91	4.53	66 %	
TLC	[L]	7.06	4.96	70 %	-3.0
VC IN	[L]	4.80	4.00	83 %	-1.4
RV	[L]	1.68	0.96	57 %	-1.8
FRC	[L]	3.29	2.25	68 %	-1.7
RV%TLC	[%]	24.49	19.28	79 %	-1.0
PaO2	[mmHg]	91			

- *Interpretation*:
  - DLCO—normal
  - KCO—normal
  - VA—normal
  - TLC—normal

Thus, it is a normal DLCO.

DIFFUSING CAPACITY FOR CARBON MONOXIDE 2

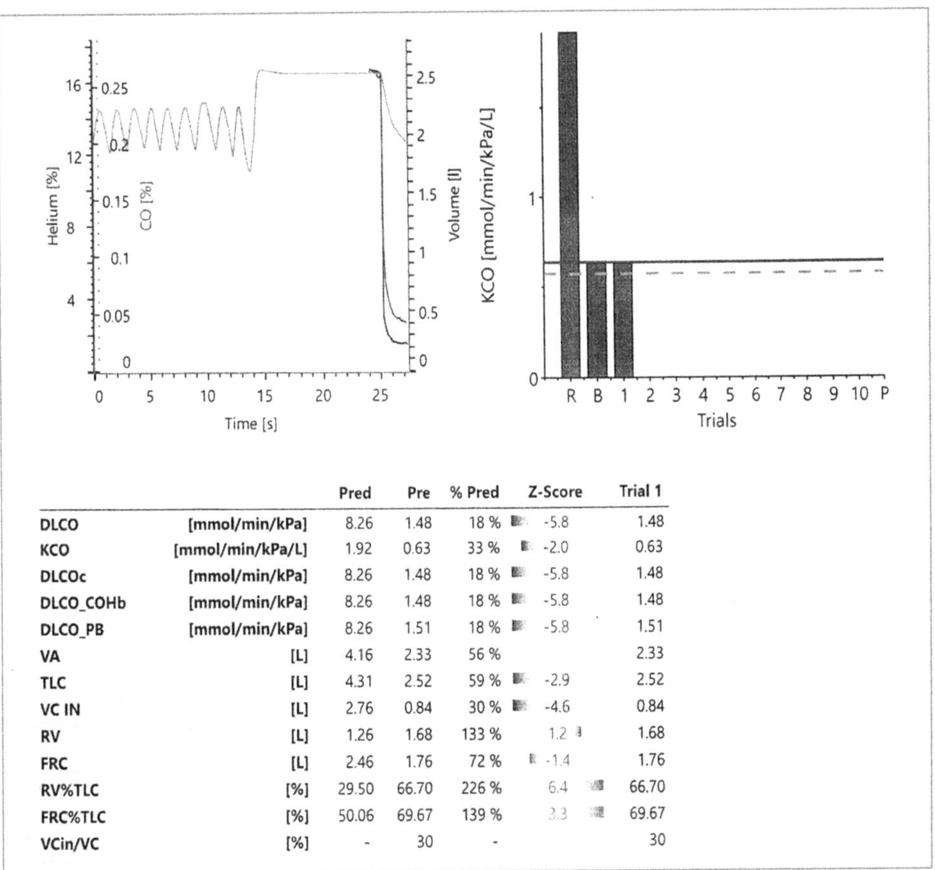

		Pred	Pre	% Pred	Z-Score	Trial 1
DLCO	[mmol/min/kPa]	8.26	1.48	18 %	-5.8	1.48
KCO	[mmol/min/kPa/L]	1.92	0.63	33 %	-2.0	0.63
DLCOc	[mmol/min/kPa]	8.26	1.48	18 %	-5.8	1.48
DLCO_COHb	[mmol/min/kPa]	8.26	1.48	18 %	-5.8	1.48
DLCO_PB	[mmol/min/kPa]	8.26	1.51	18 %	-5.8	1.51
VA	[L]	4.16	2.33	56 %		2.33
TLC	[L]	4.31	2.52	59 %	-2.9	2.52
VC IN	[L]	2.76	0.84	30 %	-4.6	0.84
RV	[L]	1.26	1.68	133 %	1.2	1.68
FRC	[L]	2.46	1.76	72 %	-1.4	1.76
RV%TLC	[%]	29.50	66.70	226 %	6.4	66.70
FRC%TLC	[%]	50.06	69.67	139 %	2.3	69.67
VCin/VC	[%]	-	30	-		30

- *Interpretation*:
  - DLCO—decreased
  - KCO—decreased
  - VA—decreased
  - TLC—decreased
- *Final impression*: Restrictive disorder

■ DIFFUSING CAPACITY FOR CARBON MONOXIDE 3

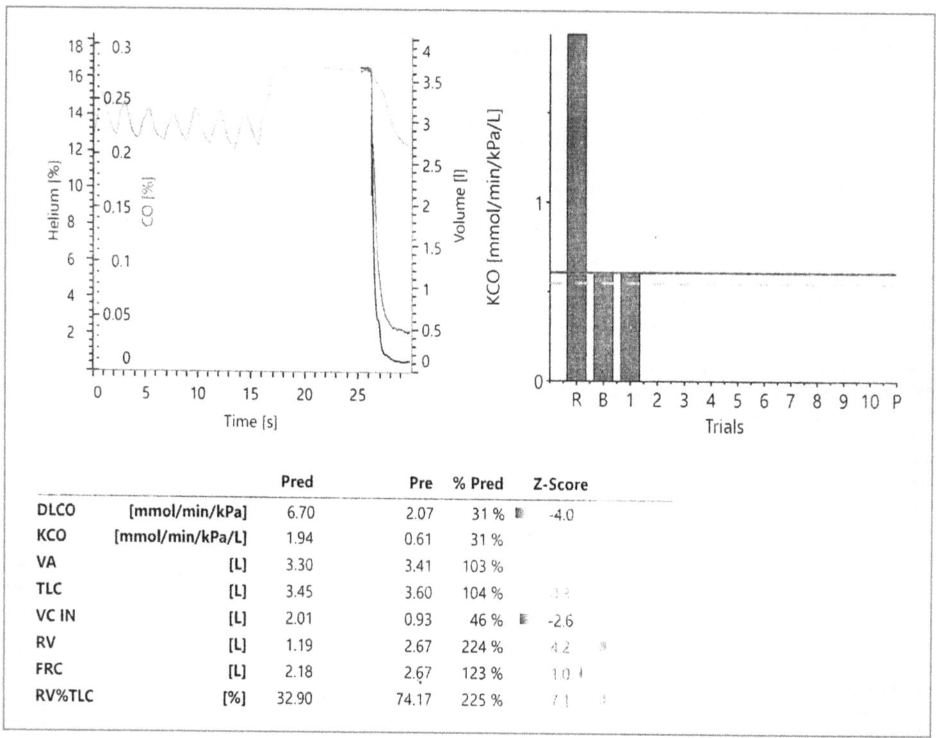

		Pred	Pre	% Pred	Z-Score
DLCO	[mmol/min/kPa]	6.70	2.07	31 %	-4.0
KCO	[mmol/min/kPa/L]	1.94	0.61	31 %	
VA	[L]	3.30	3.41	103 %	
TLC	[L]	3.45	3.60	104 %	
VC IN	[L]	2.01	0.93	46 %	-2.6
RV	[L]	1.19	2.67	224 %	
FRC	[L]	2.18	2.67	123 %	
RV%TLC	[%]	32.90	74.17	225 %	

- *Interpretation*:
  - DLCO—decreased
  - KCO—decreased
  - VA—normal
  - TLC—normal
- *Final impression*: Obstructive disorder likely emphysema.

EXERCISE

EXERCISE 1

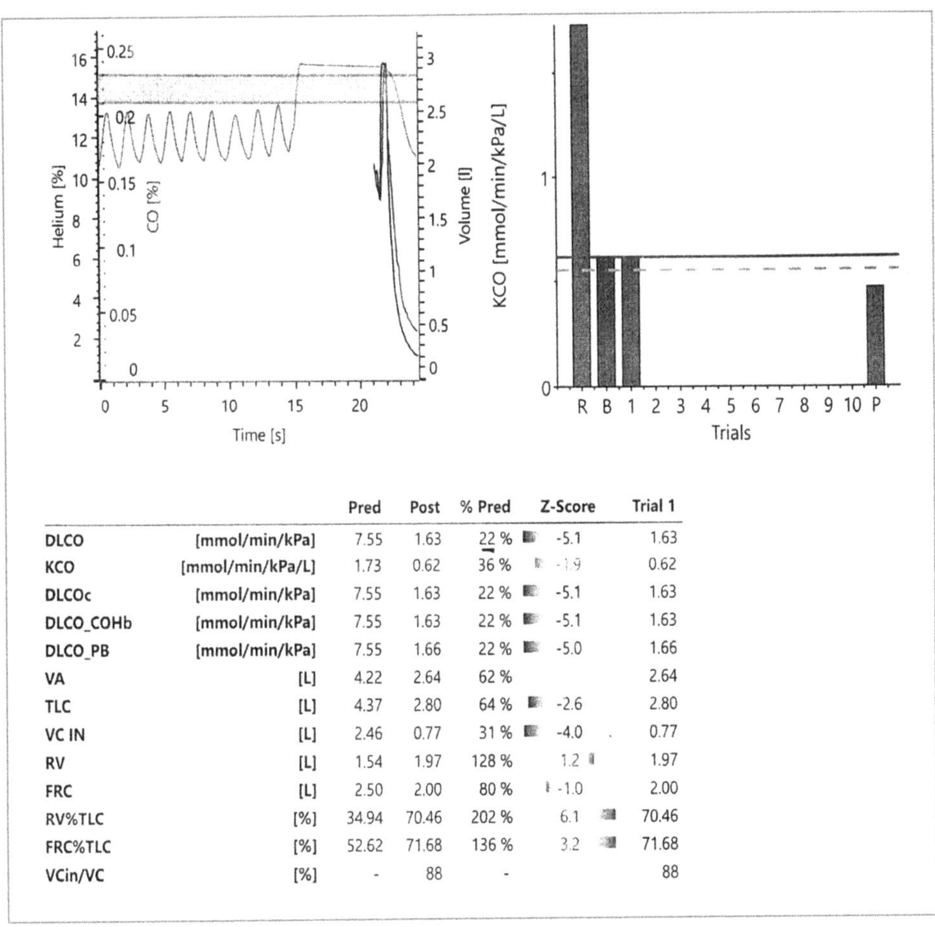

		Pred	Post	% Pred	Z-Score	Trial 1
DLCO	[mmol/min/kPa]	7.55	1.63	22 %	-5.1	1.63
KCO	[mmol/min/kPa/L]	1.73	0.62	36 %	-1.9	0.62
DLCOc	[mmol/min/kPa]	7.55	1.63	22 %	-5.1	1.63
DLCO_COHb	[mmol/min/kPa]	7.55	1.63	22 %	-5.1	1.63
DLCO_PB	[mmol/min/kPa]	7.55	1.66	22 %	-5.0	1.66
VA	[L]	4.22	2.64	62 %		2.64
TLC	[L]	4.37	2.80	64 %	-2.6	2.80
VC IN	[L]	2.46	0.77	31 %	-4.0	0.77
RV	[L]	1.54	1.97	128 %	1.2	1.97
FRC	[L]	2.50	2.00	80 %	-1.0	2.00
RV%TLC	[%]	34.94	70.46	202 %	6.1	70.46
FRC%TLC	[%]	52.62	71.68	136 %	3.2	71.68
VCin/VC	[%]	-	88	-		88

1. Interpret the DLCO.
2. Name some other conditions where you can find similar DLCO.

EXERCISE 2

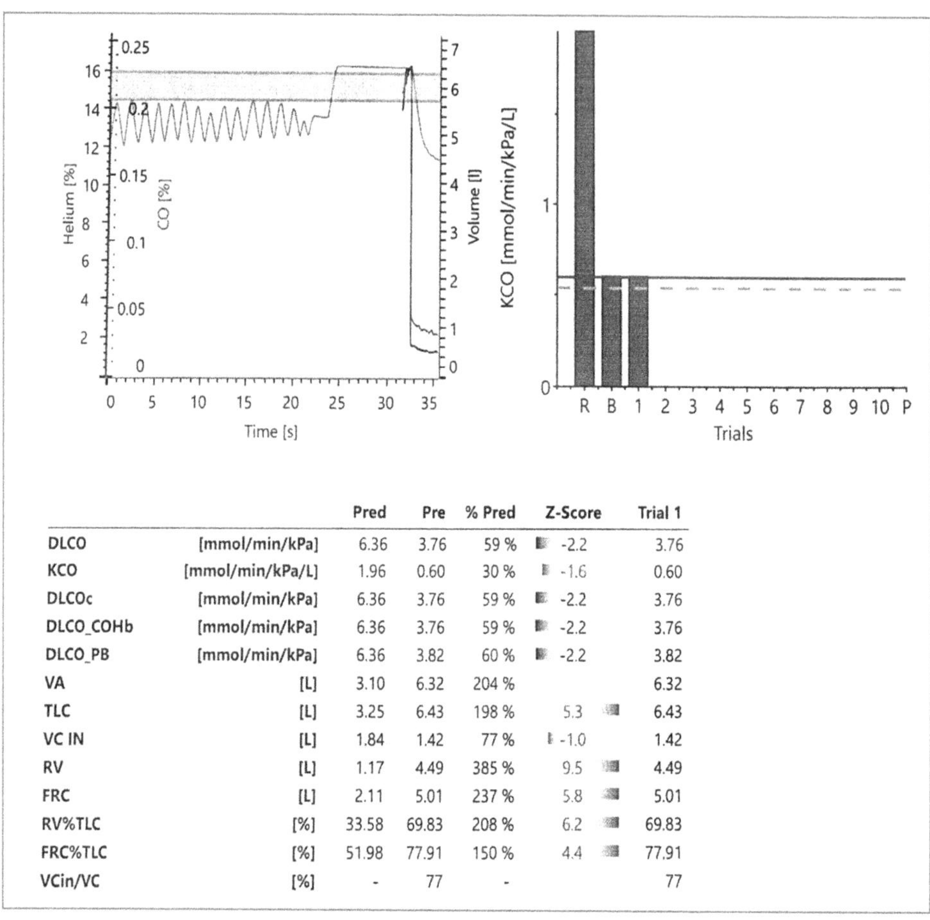

		Pred	Pre	% Pred	Z-Score	Trial 1
DLCO	[mmol/min/kPa]	6.36	3.76	59 %	-2.2	3.76
KCO	[mmol/min/kPa/L]	1.96	0.60	30 %	-1.6	0.60
DLCOc	[mmol/min/kPa]	6.36	3.76	59 %	-2.2	3.76
DLCO_COHb	[mmol/min/kPa]	6.36	3.76	59 %	-2.2	3.76
DLCO_PB	[mmol/min/kPa]	6.36	3.82	60 %	-2.2	3.82
VA	[L]	3.10	6.32	204 %		6.32
TLC	[L]	3.25	6.43	198 %	5.3	6.43
VC IN	[L]	1.84	1.42	77 %	-1.0	1.42
RV	[L]	1.17	4.49	385 %	9.5	4.49
FRC	[L]	2.11	5.01	237 %	5.8	5.01
RV%TLC	[%]	33.58	69.83	208 %	6.2	69.83
FRC%TLC	[%]	51.98	77.91	150 %	4.4	77.91
VCin/VC	[%]	-	77	-		77

1. Interpret the DLCO.
2. How will you treat the patient?

ANSWERS

EXERCISE 1

1. Interpretation
    - ↓DLCO
    - ↓KCO
    - ↓VA
    - ↓TLC

Thus, it represents a restrictive disorder.

2. Some examples of restrictive disorder are:
    - ILD
    - Chest wall deformity
    - Ankylosing spondylitis

EXERCISE 2

1. Interpretation
    - ↓DLCO
    - ↓KCO
    - ↑VA
    - ↑TLC

Thus, it represents obstructive airway disease with air trapping (↓TLC)—emphysema.

2. In case of asthma—LABA + inhaled corticosteroid (ICS). May need systemic steroids in severe cases.

    In COPD—as per 2024 Gold guidelines.
    - *Gold A*: Any bronchodilator
    - *Gold B*: LABA + long-acting muscarinic antagonist (LAMA)
    - *Gold C*: LABA + LAMA + ICS **(Fig. 16)**

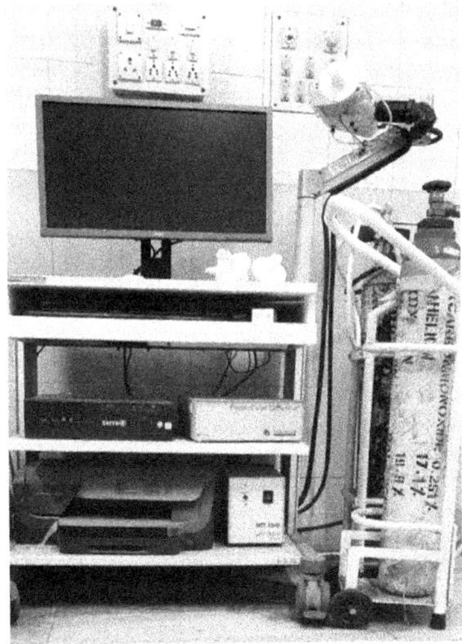

FIG. 16: A DLCO machine.

(DLCO: diffusing capacity for carbon monoxide)

HELIUM DILUTION TECHNIQUE

Helium dilution method is used to measure FRC. It is based on the equilibration of gas in the lung with a known volume of gas containing helium. The test gas consists of air, 25–30% oxygen, and 10% helium. Helium is used because it is an inert, tasteless, odorless, and nontoxic gas. It also cannot cross the alveolar-capillary membrane and is thus contained within the lungs.

Helium dilution method is done with the help of volume-displacement spirometer. The capacity of the spirometer should be 7 L. The spirometer is equipped with a mixing fan, CO_2 absorber, oxygen and helium supply, a gas inlet and a water vapor absorber in line to the helium absorber.

Procedure

- The equipment is turned on and allowed adequate time to warm-up and calibration is done.
- The procedure is explained to the patient emphasizing the need to avoid leak around the mouthpiece.
- The patient is seated comfortably, and a nose clip is applied. Ear plugs are applied if the patient has perforated ear drum.
- The patient breathes on the mouthpiece for 30–60 seconds to become accustomed to the apparatus and until a stable end-tidal expiratory level is achieved.
- The patient is turned "in", i.e., connected to the test gas at the end of normal tidal expiration.
- The patient is instructed to breathe normal tidal breaths.
- The helium concentration is noted every 15 seconds.
- When the change in helium concentration is about 0.2% for >30 seconds equilibration is considered to be achieved.
- The patient is then turned "out" once equilibration is achieved.
- At least one technically satisfactory measurement should be obtained.

The lung volume (FRCHe) at the time the subject is connected to the spirometry apparatus of a known volume (Vapp) and helium fraction (FHe1) is calculated from the helium fraction at the time of equilibration (FHe2) as follows:

$$Vapp \times FHe1 = (Vapp + FRCHe) \times FHe2$$
$$FRCHe = Vapp\ (FHe1 - FHe2)/FHe2$$

Where lung volumes include the dead space of the valve and mouthpiece, which must be subtracted, and FRCHe should be corrected to BTPS (body temperature, pressure, and saturated) conditions.

NITROGEN WASHOUT METHOD

This method is used to determine the FRC. In this method the person breathes in 100% O_2 for 7 minutes and the concentration of N2 in the expired gas is monitored. When the concentration of N2 in the expired air falls to zero, all the N2 present in the lungs at the start of O_2 breathing has been washed out. The initial N2 concentration at the start of expiration and the amount of N2 washed out is used to calculate the lung volume at the start of washout, i.e., FRC.

Procedure

- Calibration of the instrument
- The patient is seated comfortably, and the procedure is explained to the patient. There should be no leaks during washout.
- Nose clip is applied.
- The patient performs normal tidal breathing on the mouthpiece for 30–60 seconds to become accustomed to the apparatus and to assure stable end-tidal expiratory level.
- Once the breathing is stable and consistent with end-Tv at FRC, the circuit is switched on so that the patient breathes in 100% O_2.
- The N2 concentration is monitored during the washout. If there is a change in inspired N2 concentration by >0.1% or there is a sudden increase in expired N2 concentration, it indicates a leak.
- The washout is considered to be complete if the N2 concentration is 1.5% for at least three successive breaths.

The calculation of FRC is based on the assumption that volume of N2 in the lungs during the beginning of the test is the same as the volume of N2 exhaled during the test.

$$F_{ON2} \times VO = F_{EN2} \times VE$$

Where, F_{ON2} = concentration of N2 in the lungs; VO = volume of gas in the lungs; F_{EN2} = concentration of N2 in the expired gas; VE = volume of expired gas.

This volume is calculated by substituting into the above equation the initial concentration of N2 in the lungs, estimated at 0.81 in fasting and 0.79–0.80 in nonfasting subjects, and the measured values for volume and N2 concentration of expired gas.

PREOPERATIVE EVALUATION

The main components of in preoperative evaluation of surgical patients are as follows:
- History and physical examination
- Chest radiograph
- Arterial blood gas analysis
- Pulmonary function tests

History and Physical Examination

The following issues should be reviewed: (1) Smoking history, (2) history of respiratory symptoms such as cough, dyspnea, chest pain, and obstructive sleep apnea (OSA), (3) extent of pre-existing lung disease, and (4) history of respiratory tract infection.

Physical examinations are rarely helpful in identifying pulmonary risk factors. However, the initial physical examination supplements the history and provides a baseline for future comparison.

Chest Radiograph

The preoperative chest X-ray is usually unremarkable if risk factors and abnormal physical findings are absent. Screening chest X-ray is more likely to show an abnormality in individuals with known cardiopulmonary disease. Thus, a preoperative chest X-ray is useful when there are new or unexplained symptoms or signs, when there is history of underlying lung disease, and no recent chest radiography or thoracic surgery is indicated.

Arterial Blood Gas Analysis

Since an elevated pCO_2 is associated with an increased incidence of postoperative respiratory morbidity in patients with significant chronic lung disease, an arterial blood gas analysis should be done in these patients. It is common practice to obtain arterial blood gas samples in all patients undergoing lung resection surgery, irrespective of underlying lung disease.

Pulmonary Function Test

Indications for preoperative pulmonary function tests include presence of unexplained cough or dyspnea, history of chronic lung disease, a history of cigarette smoking (>20 pack years), or planned lung resection.

■ PREOPERATIVE EVALUATION FOR LUNG RESECTION

Pulmonary Function Testing

Risk of postoperative respiratory complication following pneumonectomy increases significantly when the FEV1 is <2 L or 80% of predicted normal, or when the maximal voluntary ventilation is <50% predicted. For a lobectomy, an FEV1 of 1.5 L appears to be critical threshold. The DLCO is also an important predictor of postoperative complication. Increased risk is associated with a DLCO of <60% to 80% of predicted and appears to be independent from FEV1 as a predictor of complications, morbidity and death.

Prediction of Postoperative FEV1 or DLCO

Ventilation-perfusion lung scan measures the relative blood flow or ventilation to one lung or lung region, and can be used to predict postoperative FEV1 or DLCO using the following equation:

Predicted postoperative FEV1 or DLCO = Preoperative FEV1 or DLCO × (lung function remaining after resection, as determined by radionuclide imaging)

An alternative approach to estimating the predicted postoperative pulmonary function involves a calculation based on the number of segments of the lung.

Perfusion imaging-based method provides a better prediction of postoperative lung function, as the segment method underestimates lung function after pneumonectomy.

The perioperative risk for lung resection increases significantly when the predicted postoperative FEV1 or DLCO is <40% predicted. Therefore, a predicted postoperative FEV1 or DLCO of at least 40% predicted has been proposed as useful criteria for undertaking "safe" pulmonary resection.

Exercise Testing

Measurement of maximal oxygen consumption (V_{O2MAX}) during cardiopulmonary testing is useful in predicting postoperative morbidity and mortality. Specifically, a V_{O2MAX} of

<15–20 mL/kg/min is associated with an increased incidence of postoperative complications. Cardiopulmonary exercise testing is therefore used to further assess the operability of patients who would be at a high risk for surgery based on determination of predicted postoperative pulmonary function.

If cardiopulmonary exercise testing is unavailable, two simpler tests, stair climbing and a walking test, can be used to assess a patient's fitness for lung resection.

A patient's ability to climb five flights of stairs predicts a V_{O2MAX} >20 mL/kg/min. Patients who are unable to climb one flight of stairs have a V_{O2MAX} <10 mL/kg/min. An ability to climb three flights of stairs reliably identifies patients who are likely to do well after a lobectomy, despite having a predicted postoperative FEV1 or DLCO, that is <40% of predicted.

The shuttle walk and 6-minute walk test are also important alternatives to cardiopulmonary exercise testing. For the shuttle walk, the patient walks back and forth over a distance of 25 m at a progressively faster rate. Inability to complete 25 shuttles approximates a V_{O2MAX} <10 mL/kg/min. A 6-minute walk distance >1,000 ft has been reported as predictive of successful surgical outcome.

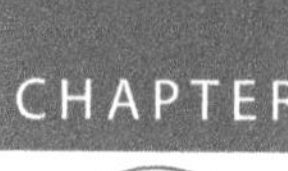

Polysomnography

Saikat Banerjee

INTRODUCTION

Sleep has remained a mysterious and interesting topic for mankind for ages. It has been mentioned in the old Hindu texts, Vedas, Upanishads, Christian Bible, and Islamic text Quran to name a few. In modern times, even though we have come a long way and are now using many sophisticated methods to understand sleep, it remains an enigmatic field with answers still waiting to be found.

In the modern era, we have realized that the understanding of sleep can be achieved by monitoring the functioning of vital body systems such as nervous, respiratory, circulatory, gastrointestinal, musculoskeletal, endocrinal, and genitourinary systems. This is because the activity of these systems varies markedly in wakefulness and sleep states. It is for this reason that the simultaneous recording of electroencephalogram (EEG), electrooculogram (EOG), electromyogram (EMG), electrocardiogram (ECG), respiratory movements of thorax and abdomen, nasal airflow, nasal air pressure, nasal and labial (lip) temperature (recorded by thermistor) is done to monitor, screen, and diagnose sleep disorders. The term polysomnography (PSG) is the term used to describe this procedure ("poly"—many, "somno"—sleep, and "graphy"—recording procedure).

Sleep disorders can broadly be divided into dyssomnias (disturbances in the amount, quality, or timing of sleep) and parasomnias (dysfunctional or episodic events occurring in sleep). The International Classification of Sleep Disorders, 3rd edition (ICSD-3) classifies sleep disorders into insomnias (reduction in the quantity/duration of sleep), sleep-related breathing disorders (SRBDs), central disorders of hypersomnolence (increase in sleep quantity), circadian rhythm sleep-wake disorders, parasomnias, sleep-related movement disorders (SRMDs), and other miscellaneous sleep disorders.

In the eyes of a respiratory physician, the greatest emphasis is put on SRBDs only, as will be the case for this chapter too; however, a sleep physician should develop mastery over all the above disorders that have been mentioned.

INDICATIONS AND TYPES OF POLYSOMNOGRAPHY

A sleep study or a PSG is done for diagnostic, titration (therapeutic), or follow-up purposes. Any patient with a differential diagnosis that includes a sleep disorder should preferably undergo a diagnostic nocturnal PSG. Symptoms such as excessive daytime sleepiness, choking during sleep, witnessed apneas, snoring, daytime fatigue, and loss of alertness with or without the presence of cardiovascular and endocrine abnormalities raise the suspicion of a sleep disorder. Nowadays, some surrogate methods such as home sleep apnea testing (HSAT) or out-of-center sleep testing (OCST), actigraphy watches, sleep pillows, and smart watches using cardioballistograms are also being used to detect sleep disorders, but PSG remains the test of choice for diagnosing SRBDs.

Based on the number of parameters being monitored in PSG, it is divided into four types: Type 1, which is a fully attended PSG with ≥7 channels; Type 2, a fully unattended study with ≥7 channels; Type 3, unattended limited channel study with 4–7 channels; and Type 4, unattended study with 1 or 2 channels using oximetry as one of the parameters. A type 1 or a type 2 PSG is recommended for diagnosis of SRBDs.

The PSG is usually done as a continuous nocturnal overnight study as a diagnostic study or a therapeutic titration study [with continuous positive airway pressure (CPAP) or bi-level positive airway pressure (BiPAP), which is the main treatment for SRBDs]. In cases with severe sleep disorders, diagnostic and therapeutic studies can be done in a single night called split-night studies. Finally, in special cases, we can perform daytime PSGs, like in night-shift workers or sleep latency tests for insomnia and narcolepsy.

We will not focus on the attachments involved in a PSG study or the patient preparations required in this chapter. However, the reader is urged to read further and understand the electronics involved, the principles underlying the PSG channels, and the preparations involved in conducting the study.

In this chapter, we will first learn to identify sleep stages in a PSG. Subsequently, we will learn to identify apneas (central, obstructive, and mixed), hypopneas (central and obstructive), sleep-related hypoxemia, and hypoventilation events using the present American Academy of Sleep Medicine (AASM) guidelines.

LEARNING OBJECTIVES

1. To learn the importance of and an overview of the principles of polysomnography.
2. To understand the indications of polysomnography.
3. To learn to interpret and diagnose stages of sleep.
4. To learn to interpret basic sleep graphs pertaining to common sleep-related breathing disorders.

UNDERSTANDING THE CHANNELS IN POLYSOMNOGRAPHY TRACING

Before moving any further, we will first understand the channels which are shown in a polysomnograph. The first six channels usually depict the EEG recording. Two channels each from frontal (F3 and F4), parietal (C3 and C4), and occipital lobes (O1 and O2) are used, one of them being the backup. They are recorded against reference electrodes placed on the mastoid (M1, M2, or A1, A2). Accordingly, the EEG channels are labeled F3M2 (F3A2), F4M1 (F4A1), C3M2 (C3A2), C4M1 (C4A1), O1M2 (O1A2), and O2M1 (O2A1). The important point to remember is that even numbering is used for right-sided leads and odd numbering for left-sided leads.

For EOG the channels are named EOG2A2 (or EOG2M2) and EOG1A2 (or EOG1M2). Other names might be LEOG and REOG in place of EOG1 and EOG2, respectively. Note that EOG leads are referenced from a single mastoid electrode unlike EEG leads. This is done to capture conjugate movements of the eyes (movements of both eyes are interrelated).

The EMG channels are usually labeled EMG or Chin EMG. Sometimes, there are two channels EMG1 and EMG2. If limb leads for recording leg movements during sleep are placed, they are usually labeled periodic limb movement (PLM)1 and PLM2. Apart from this impedance, pulse transit time (PTT), body plethysmography (body pleth), and ECG channels are also usually present. Channels for respiratory parameters will be discussed briefly when we will discuss the interpretation of respiratory events during sleep.

CONCEPT OF THE EPOCH

A standard overnight PSG usually is 6–8 hours long. During this, there are several respiratory events and numerous transitions between various stages of sleep. It is impossible to analyze such huge data with so much variation just at a single glance, neither is it possible to be fitted into a single screen for the same. Hence, we need to break up this data into small parts and analyze each part separately for events during sleep and also staging of sleep. Each such part is termed an epoch. The duration of the epoch, however, is variable. During sleep staging the epoch used is of 30-second duration, for respiratory events, it is of 2 minutes duration, 5 minutes for Cheyne–Stokes breathing and leg movements, and 15 seconds each for seizures and ECG. The timing of the epochs has been optimized as mentioned earlier depending on what parameter is being scored.

IDENTIFYING SLEEP STAGES

The primary goal in the interpretation of a sleep graph is to first identify the sleep stage. Needless to mention, we would generally not score any sleep events if we identified that the patient was awake during that period. In a PSG, we have the following markers for staging sleep: W for the awake state, N1, N2, and N3 for stages of nonrapid-eye-movement (NREM) sleep, and R for rapid eye movement (REM) sleep. Note that this chapter will not cover sleep staging rules exhaustively, and will cover only sleep stage identification in adults, hence, the enthusiastic reader is suggested to read the latest AASM sleep scoring manual for the details of the same.

General Principles

The 30-second epochs are used to score sleep stages. A single epoch is assigned a single stage, however, if two or more stages coexist in the same epoch, we need to identify the epoch having the sleep stage which comprises the greatest portion of it (meaning, for >15 seconds).

Following are the definitions for EEG waves: Slow wave activity is defined as a frequency of 0.5–2.0 Hz and peak-to-peak amplitude of >75 μV, measured over the frontal regions. Delta waves are defined as 0–3.99 Hz (frontal and parietal regions), theta waves as 4–7.99 Hz, alpha waves are 8–13 Hz (occipital regions), and beta waves as greater than 13 Hz.

Identifying the Wake Stage

The wake stage is identified when the following are present in the majority of a sleep epoch of 30 seconds:

- *Presence of alpha rhythm:* A train of sinusoidal 8–13 Hz EEG activity recorded over the occipital regions.
- *Eye blinks:* Presence of conjugate vertical eye movements with eyes open or closed with a frequency of 0.5–2 Hz.
- *Reading eye movements:* Eye movement occurs in the opposite direction as the reading of the person. Consists of slow and rapid phase conjugate eye movements.
- *Rapid eye movements:* Irregular, conjugate, and sharp-peaked eye movements with initial eye deflection <500 ms. This is also seen in REM sleep.
- *Slow eye movements (SEMs):* Regular, sinusoidal, and conjugate eye movements with initial deflection >500 ms. This may be seen in the wake stage with eyes closed or in the N1 stage.

Wake stage criteria are thus the following (1 and/or 2):

1. Predominant alpha rhythm in the majority of the epoch.
2. *Other findings consistent with wake stage:* Eye blinks, REMs with high chin-EMG tone, and reading eye movements.
   A classic example of the wake stage is given in **Figure 1**.

Identifying N1 Stage

For the N1 stage, we need to learn the following terms:

- *Low-amplitude mixed frequency (LAMF) waves in EEG:* Predominant EEG activity in the range of 4–7 Hz. EEG activity is slower than at least 1 Hz from what is observed in the wake stage.

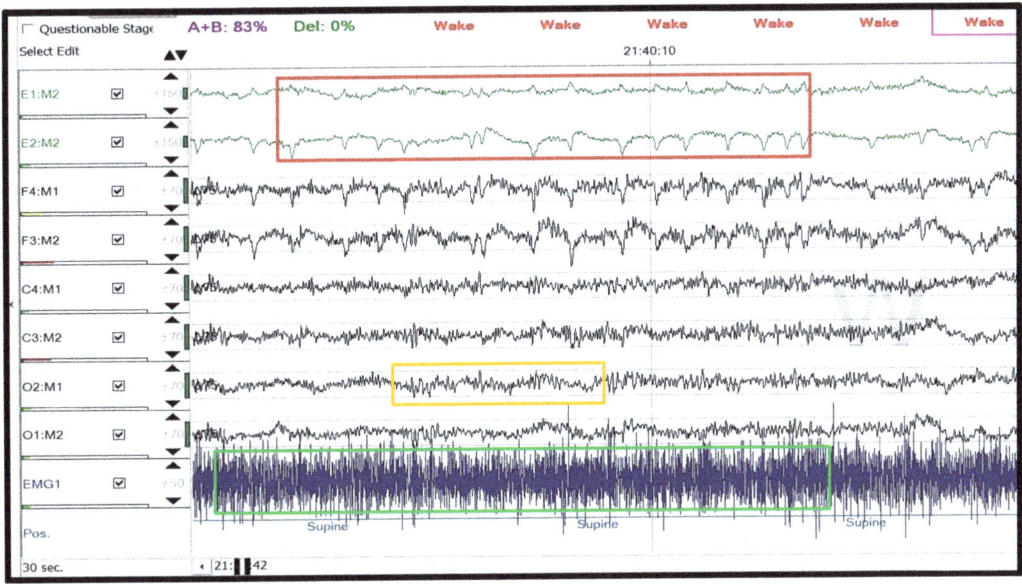

FIG. 1: Wake stage [alpha waves (yellow box), reading eye movements, and blinks (red box), high electromyogram (EMG) tone (green box)].

Note: The time when the patient is disconnected from the recording equipment is also scored as the wake stage.

- *Vertex sharp waves (V waves):* May occur in both N1 and N2 sleep but commonly occur in the transition to N1 stage of sleep. They are sharply contoured waves with peaks over the central region with a duration of <0.5 seconds (measured at the base of the wave).
- *Sleep onset:* It is a term used for the start of the first epoch scored as any stage of sleep (usually, it is N1).

Score and epoch as N1 stage if any of the following are satisfied:
- Presence of LAMF EEG activity in >50% of the epoch.
- Presence of vertex waves.
- SEMs present >50% of the epoch.

As long as there is no evidence for another sleep stage, the subsequent epochs are also scored as N1. If during sleep stages other than N1 (N2, N3, or R), arousal occurs and is followed by LAMF (and also SEM should be present if the previous epoch was REM sleep), then that epoch shall be scored as the N1 stage.

Figure 2 shows an example of stage N1 sleep.

Identifying N2 Stage

The following definitions are important for scoring the N2 stage:
1. *K complex:* A characteristic wave seen with maximal amplitude in frontal EEG derivations, which has an initial sharp negative deflection followed by a positive component and stands out from the background EEG with a total duration of ≥0.5 seconds. An arousal is said to be associated with a K complex when it occurs within one second of its termination.
2. *Sleep spindle:* These are a series of waves with a crescendo-decrescendo pattern (like a spindle) and frequency between 11 and 16 Hz and duration of ≥0.5 seconds. These waves are maximal in amplitude in central EEG derivations.

Score a stage as N2 if in the first half of an epoch or the last half of the previous epoch, either one or more K complexes without any associated arousal are present; or there are sleep spindles **(Fig. 3)**.

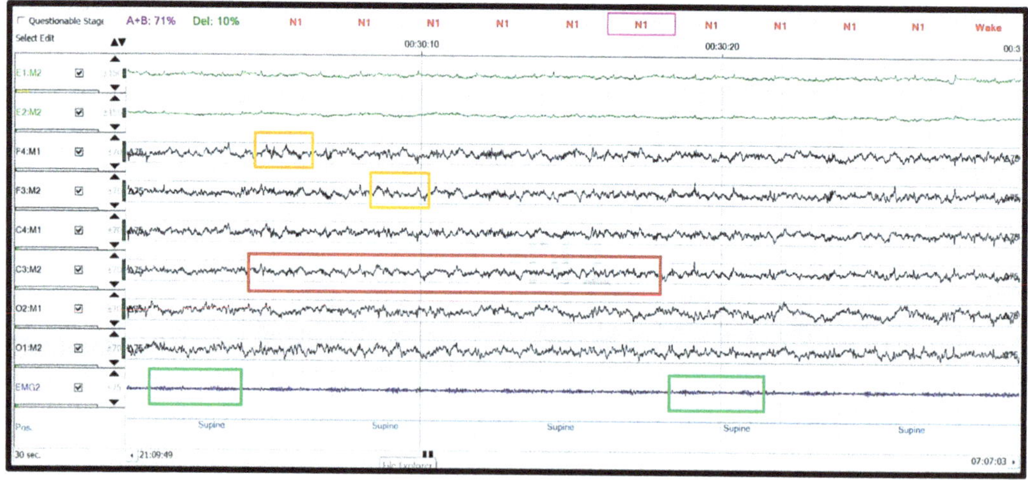

FIG. 2: N1 stage of sleep [vertex waves in groups (yellow boxes), low-amplitude mixed frequency EEG activity (red box), and low chin EMG tone as compared to wake stage (green boxes)].

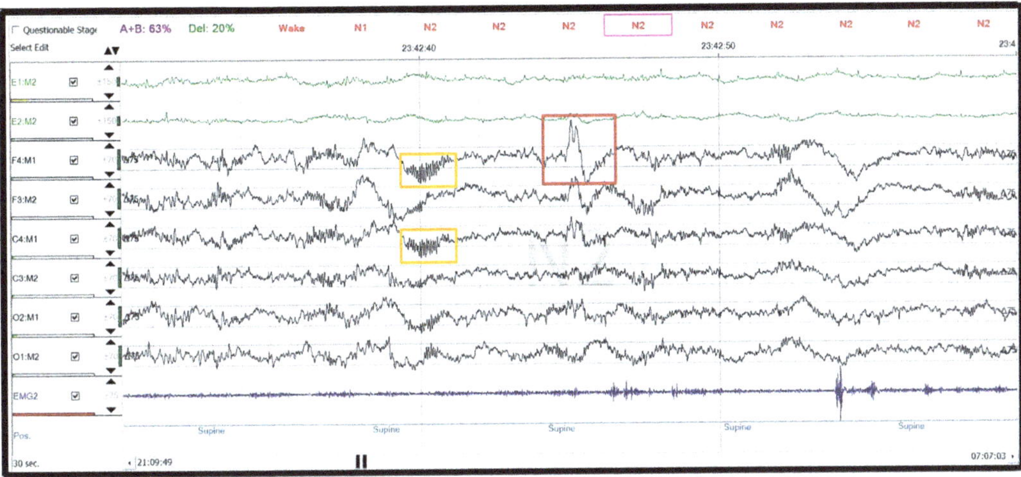

FIG. 3: N2 stage of sleep showing sleep spindles (yellow boxes) and K complexes (red box).

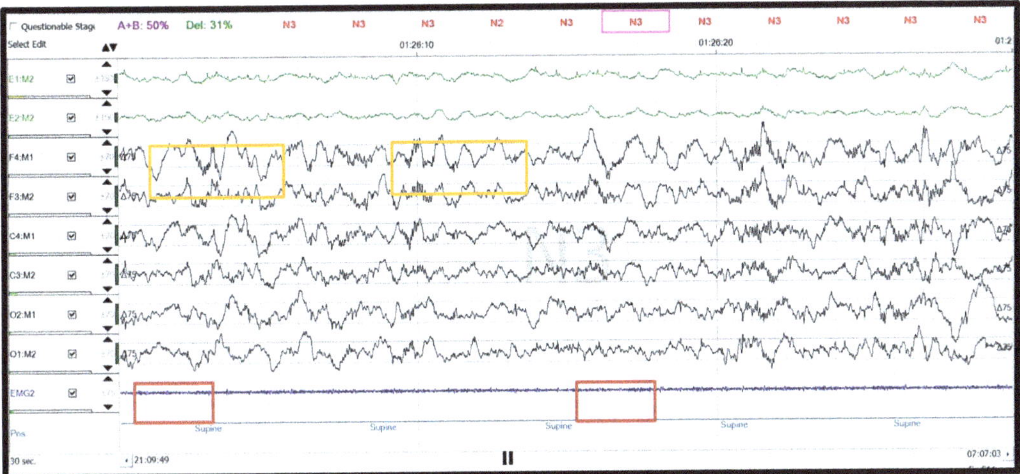

FIG. 4: N3 stage of sleep, showing slow wave activity (yellow boxes), and low chin tone in EMG (red boxes).

Scoring of the N2 stage is ended in any of the following cases:
- Transition to stage N3, R, or W stage.
- An arousal followed by LAMF and SEM, in such case it will be scored as N1.
- A major body movement followed by LAMF and SEM, also scored as N1.

Identifying N3 Stage

The N3 is defined by slow wave activity occurring in ≥20% of the epoch (≥6 seconds). Slow wave activity refers to EEG waves ranging from 0.5 to 2 Hz (in the delta range) and peak-to-peak amplitude of >75 μV measured over the frontal derivations **(Fig. 4)**.

Special considerations include the following:
- K complexes may be considered as slow waves if they meet the criteria for slow wave activity.
- Sleep spindles may be present in N3 sleep.
- Eye movements are not seen in N3 sleep usually.
- Chin EMG tone is low, even sometimes as low as in REM sleep.

Identifying R Stage

The following are the specific findings in REM sleep:
- *Rapid eye movements:* Conjugate, irregular, sharp, and peaked movements of the eye with initial deflection lasting <500 ms present in the EOG derivations are termed REMs. They can be seen both in the wake and REM sleep stages.
- *Low chin EMG tone:* The chin EMG levels are lowest at this level of sleep.
- *Sawtooth waves:* Serrated and sharply contoured, train of triangular waves with a frequency of 2–6 Hz occurring in maximal amplitude over central head regions and may sometimes precede a burst of REMs.
- *Transient muscle activity:* Bursts of EMG activity <0.25 seconds superimposed on low EMG tone seen in the chin EMG or PLM leads as well as sometimes in the EEG or EOG derivations. Such activity may be found in high amplitude when associated with REMs.

An epoch is scored as REM sleep (definite stage R) if all of the following are satisfied:
- LAMF without K complexes or sleep spindles.
- Low chin EMG tone for the majority of epoch and concurrent with REMs.
- REMs at any position within the epoch.

All epochs preceding and after an epoch of definite stage R are scored as REM sleep if the following criteria are met:
- EEG shows LAMF without any sleep spindles or K complexes.
- The chin EMG is low (at stage R level).
- No intervening arousal
- SEMs following an arousal or stage W are absent.
  Figure 5 shows a 30-second PSG epoch of REM sleep.

Scoring of stage R should be ended in the following cases:
- In cases of transition to stage W, N3, or N2.
- In cases of increase in chin EMG tone and meeting criteria for N1, or if there is an arousal/major body movement followed by LAMF and SEM.

Arousal rule: Score arousal in stages N1, N2, N3, or R in case of abrupt shift in frequencies to >16 Hz lasting for at least 3 seconds with ≥10 seconds of stable sleep preceding the event.

Major body movement: It is a movement and muscle artifact that obscures the EEG to such an extent that an exact sleep stage cannot be scored.

IDENTIFYING RESPIRATORY EVENTS

To identify respiratory events in PSG, it is important to study the airflow and body movements. The following PSG channels in order of preference are used to monitor the airflow for apneas:
- Oronasal thermistor

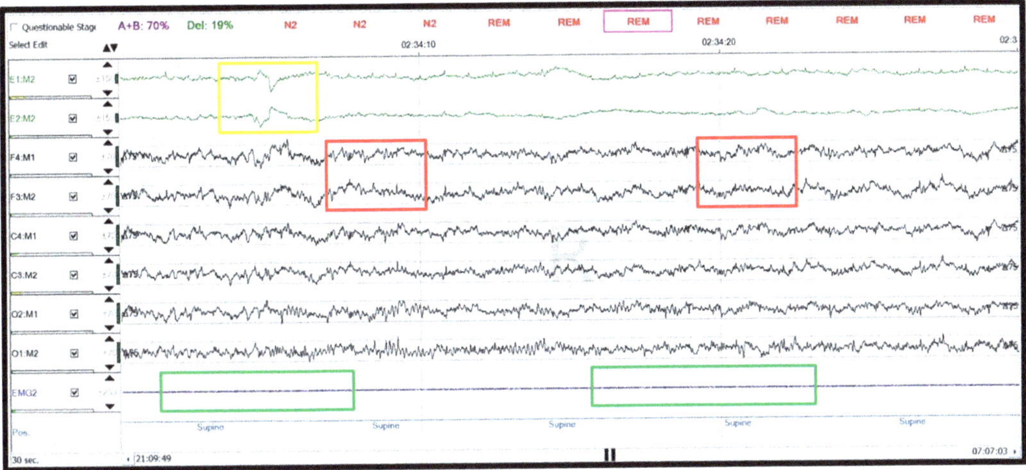

FIG. 5: REM sleep stage showing rapid eye movement (yellow box), sawtooth waves (red boxes), and low to absent chin EMG tone (green boxes).

- Nasal pressure transducer
- Respiratory inductance plethysmography sum (RIPsum)
- Respiratory inductance plethysmography flow (thorax or abdomen) (RIPflow)
- Polyvinylidene fluoride impedance sensor (PVDFsum)

The following PSG channels in order of preference are used to monitor the airflow for hypopneas:
- Nasal pressure transducer
- Oronasal thermistor
- RIPsum
- RIPflow (thorax or abdomen)
- Dual thoracoabdominal RIP belts
- PVDFsum

For titration studies, a positive airway pressure (PAP) device flow signal should be used to identify apneas or hypopneas. The following PSG channels in order of preference are used to monitor respiratory efforts:
- Esophageal manometry
- Dual thoracoabdominal RIP belts
- Dual thoracoabdominal PVDFsum belts

There are separate sensors for monitoring the oxygen saturation (pulse oximeter) and snoring (acoustic sensor, piezoelectric sensor, or may be recorded by nasal pressure transducer). For detection of hypoventilation, arterial, transcutaneous, or end-tidal (only during the diagnostic study) pCO_2 is recommended.

To measure the duration of any respiratory event, the measurement is taken from the nadir preceding the first breath which is reduced to the beginning of the first breath that reaches close to the baseline amplitude.

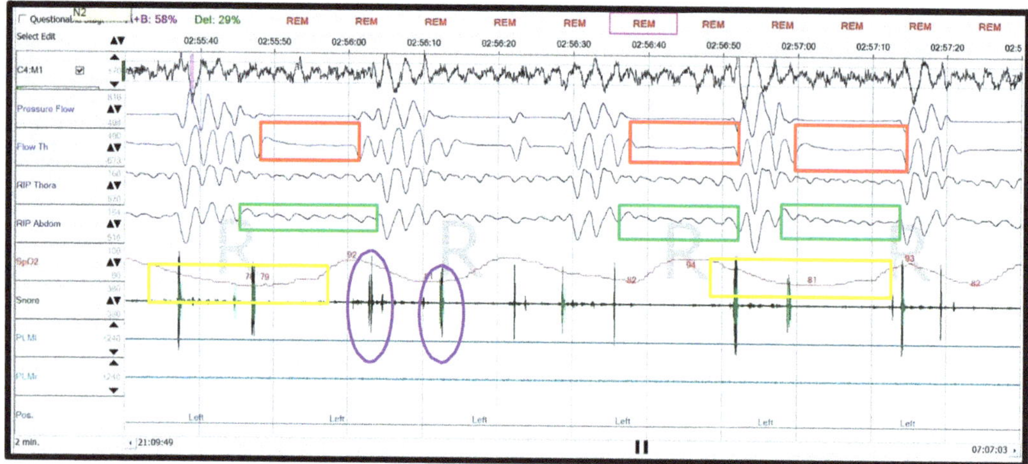

FIG. 6: PSG showing obstructive sleep apnea: Red boxes indicating absent flow in thermistor, green boxes showing decreased (but not absent) respiratory efforts, yellow boxes showing desaturation during the event, and purple circles indicating the presence of snoring during and after the event.

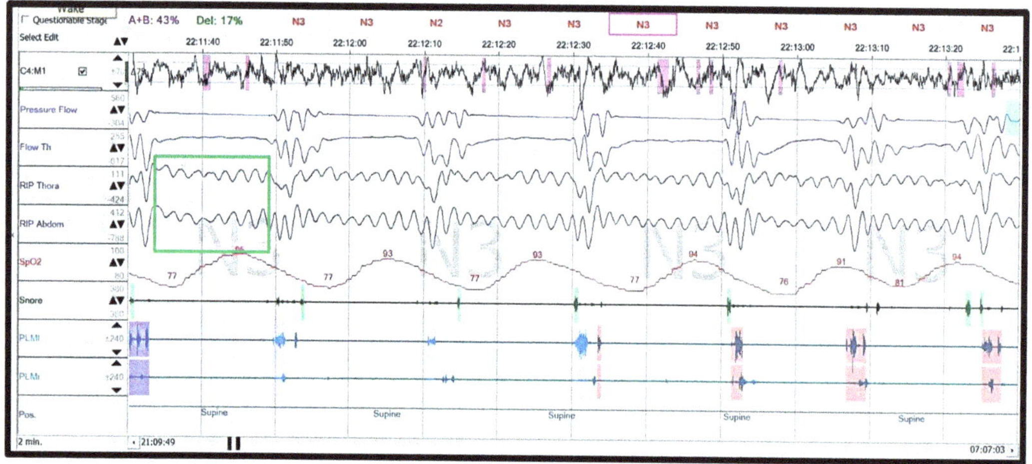

FIG. 7: Another example of obstructive sleep apnea showing paradoxical thoracoabdominal respiration (green box showing downstroke of abdominal movement coinciding with upstroke of thoracic movement). Also, note that the epoch for respiratory events is set at 2 minutes.

Scoring Apneas

The following criteria are needed to identify a respiratory event as apnea:

- Reduction in peak signal intensity by ≥90% from the pre-event baseline using any of the recommended sensors.
- The duration of this reduction should be ≥10 seconds.

Obstructive apnea is identified when apnea is associated with continuous or increased inspiratory effort in the absence of airflow **(Fig. 6)**. A paradoxical movement of the thorax and abdomen may also be observed in some cases **(Fig. 7)**.

Central apnea is identified when apnea is associated with the absence of inspiratory effort in the period of absent airflow **(Fig. 8)**. Central sleep apneas (CSAs) are disorders having predominantly central apnea events and are classified into a variety of types including Cheyne's Stokes breathing, CSA due to medical disorder, high-altitude periodic breathing, medication or substance use, primary CSA, and primary CSA in infancy and prematurity. In some cases, CSA also appears after treatment of sleep disorders with CPAP therapy or surgical interventions. In such cases, the term treatment-emergent CSA (TECSA) is used. Mixed apnea is identified when apnea is associated with absent inspiratory effort in the initial part of the event followed by the presence of inspiratory effort in the later part of the event **(Fig. 9)**.

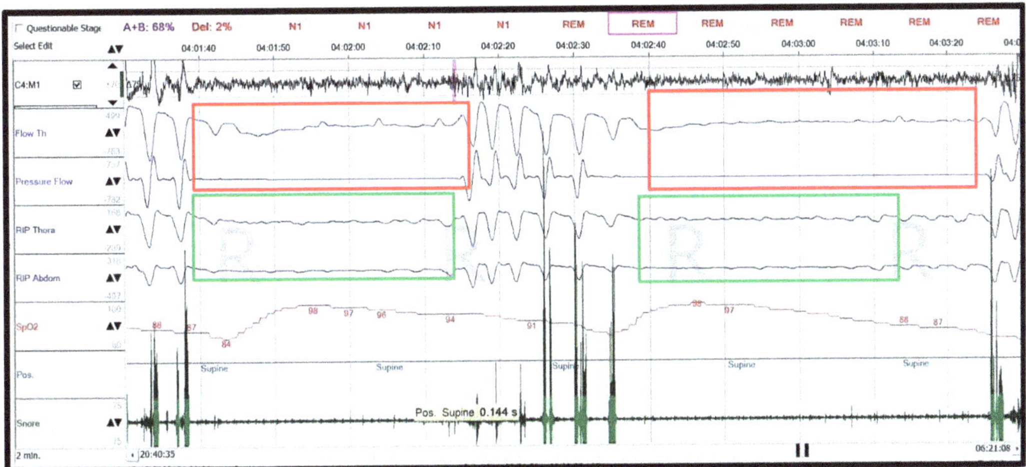

FIG. 8: Absence of or >90% decrement in signals in flow thermistor and pressure flow sensors (red boxes) indicating apnea. Also, there is a loss of respiratory effort (green boxes) indicating central apnea.

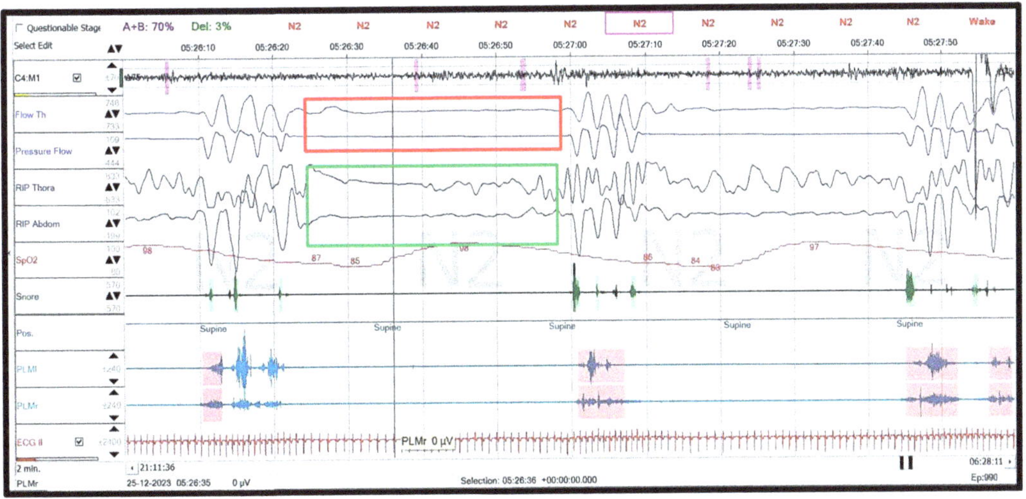

FIG. 9: An event of mixed apnea, where there is no signal in both flow thermistor and nasal pressure transducer (red box) with respiratory efforts absent in the initial part of the event but some respiratory efforts appear in the later part of the event (green box). This indicates the initial part of the event behaves like central apnea and the later part as obstructive apnea.

Scoring Hypopneas

The following criteria are needed to identify a respiratory event as hypopnea:
- Reduction in peak signal intensity by ≥30% but <90% from the pre-event baseline using any of the recommended sensors.
- The duration of this reduction should be ≥10 seconds.
- There should be either a desaturation of ≥3% from baseline or the event should be associated with an arousal.

Obstructive hypopneas **(Fig. 10)** are identified by association of hypopnea with any of the following:
- Presence of snoring during the event.
- Increased inspiratory flattening of the nasal pressure transducer or PAP device flow signal (in titration study).
- Associated thoracoabdominal paradox occurring during the event but not in pre-event breaths.

The absence of all the above criteria for obstructive hypopnea is the identification criteria for central hypopnea **(Fig. 11)**.

IDENTIFYING RESPIRATORY EFFORT-RELATED AROUSALS

Respiratory effort-related arousals (RERA) is an event with a sequence of breaths with a duration of ≥10 seconds, where either there is increasing inspiratory effort, flattening of the inspiratory portion of nasal pressure, or flattening of PAP device flow leading to an arousal from sleep but that which does not meet the criteria for apnea or hypopnea.

Obstructive sleep apnea (OSA) is a disorder characterized by classical symptoms and obstructive apneas, hypopnea, and RERA events ≥5 per hour for adults (or ≥15 per hour even without any symptoms) and ≥1 per hour for children. The classification of OSAs thus includes adult and pediatric OSA.

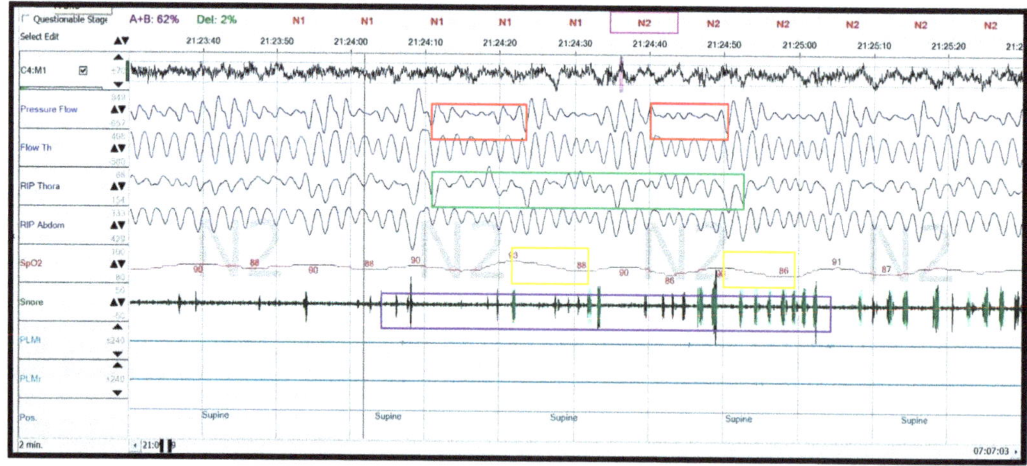

FIG. 10: Example of obstructive hypopnea: Red boxes show a reduction in signals in nasal pressure flow of > 30% with preserved respiratory efforts throughout the events (green box). Desaturation of >3% is seen in both the events (yellow boxes) with associated snoring (purple box). Note that in respiratory event scoring the topmost channel is that of EEG (C4M1) lead, as the presence and absence of arousals are also important to detect hypopnea.

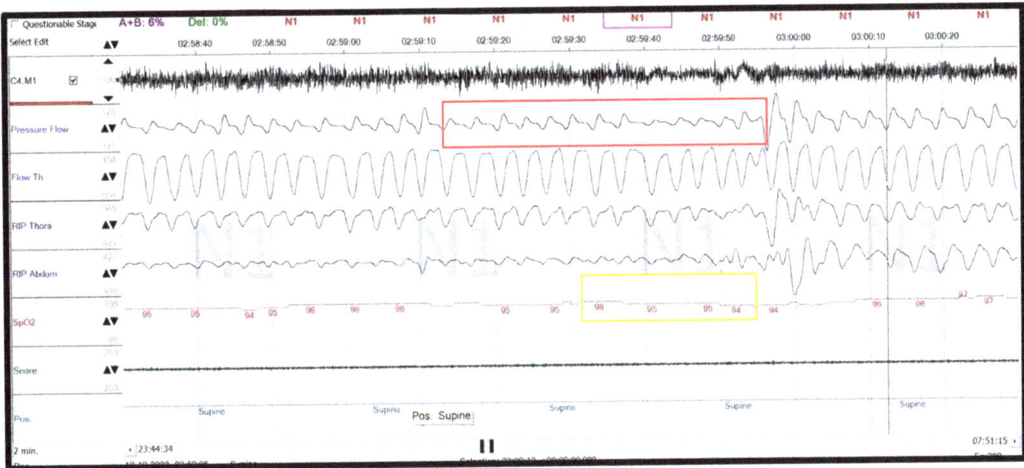

FIG. 11: A not-so-common event of central hypopnea, with reduced signal intensity in nasal pressure flow (red box), presence of normal thoracic and abdominal movements without any paradox, absence of snoring, no inspiratory airflow flattening, but with desaturation of 3% (from 96 to 93%, yellow box).

IDENTIFYING SLEEP-RELATED HYPOVENTILATION

It is important to note that the monitoring of hypoventilation during sleep is optional. Nevertheless, sleep-related hypoventilation is identified by any one of the following criteria:

- Increase in arterial pCO_2 or surrogate measurement to a value of >55 mm Hg for ≥10 minutes.
- Increase of ≥10 mm Hg in arterial pCO_2 or surrogate during sleep as compared to awake supine value or an absolute value of >50 mm Hg for ≥10 minutes.

Overall sleep-related hypoventilation disorders are of various types including obesity hypoventilation syndrome (OHS), late-onset central hypoventilation with hypothalamic dysfunction [now called rapid-onset obesity with hypothalamic dysfunction, hypoventilation, and autonomic dysregulation (ROHHAD) syndrome], idiopathic central alveolar hypoventilation, congenital central alveolar hypoventilation (CCHS, Ondine's curse), sleep hypoventilation related to a medical disorder and substance abuse. We encourage the readers to explore further and read about these disorders which we will not be covering in this chapter.

IDENTIFYING SLEEP-RELATED HYPOXEMIA

Sleep-related hypoxemia is defined as a condition where oxygen saturation is ≤88% during sleep for at least 5 minutes without hypoventilation or any other SRBD. Miscellaneous sleep disorders such as snoring and catathrenia are other SRBDs, which may be present in isolation and sometimes may be normal variants as well.

ACKNOWLEDGMENT

I would like to express my heart-felt gratitude to Dr Krishnapriya S Kumar, for providing with the sleep graphs for completion of this chapter.

Suggested Readings

While this chapter covers the basic sleep graphs that are encountered in SRBDs, it does not cover all the rules essential for sleep scoring. It also does not cover the diagnostic criteria or management of the above disorders. The following books and articles are recommended for further reading to enrich the knowledge of the rapidly expanding field of sleep medicine.

1. AASM. (2024). AASM scoring Manual Version 3. [online] Available from https://members. aasm.org/site/AASMMembers/AASMStore/StoreLayouts/Item_Detail.aspx?iProd uctCode=2100V3E&Category=CLINIC_RES. [Last accessed September, 2024].

2. AASM. The International Classification of Sleep Disorders: (ICSD-3), 3rd edition. Darien Illinois: Am Acad Sleep Med; 2014.

3. Berry RB, Quan SF, Abreu AR, Bibbs ML, DelRosso L, Harding SM, et al. The AASM Manual for the scoring of sleep and associated events: Rules, terminology and technical specifications. Darien, Ilinois: Am Acad Sleep Med; 2020.

4. AASM. International Classification of Sleep Disorders ICSD-3-text revision. Darien, Illinois: Am Acad Sleep Med; 2023.

5. Berry RB, Wagner MH. Sleep medicine pearls: Expert consult – online, 3rd edition. London: Elsevier Health Sciences; 2014.

6. Berry RB. Fundamentals of Sleep Medicine, 1st edition. Philadelphia, Pa: Elsevier Saunders; 2012.

7. Kryger MH, Rosenberg R, Kirsch DB. Kryger's sleep medicine review: A problem-oriented approach, 3rd edition. Philadelphia, PA: Elsevier; 2020.

8. Kryger MH, Roth T, Goldstein CA, Dement WC. Principles and practice of Sleep Medicine, 7th edition. Philadelphia, PA: Elsevier; 2022.

9. Kushida CA, Chediak A, Berry RB, Brown LK, Gozal D, Iber C, et al. Clinical guidelines for the manual titration of positive airway pressure in patients with obstructive sleep apnea. J Clin Sleep Med. 2008;4(2):157-71.

10. Ramírez Molina RI, Pépin J-L, Masa Jiménez JF. Obesity hypoventilation syndrome. ERS Handbook Respir Sleep Med. 2023;254-62.

11. BaHammam AS, Singh T, George S, Acosta KL, Barataman K, Gacuan DE. Choosing the right interface for positive airway pressure therapy in patients with obstructive sleep apnea. Sleep Breath. 2017;21(3):569-75.

Index

Page numbers followed by *f* refer to figure, *fc* refer to flowchart, and *t* refer to table.

EU GSPR Authorised Reprsentative
Logos Europe, 9 rue Nicolas Poussin
1700, La Rochelle, France
Phone: +33 (0) 6 67 93 73 78
E-mail: contact@logoseurope.eu

www.ingramcontent.com/pod-product-compliance
Ingram Content Group UK Ltd.
Pitfield, Milton Keynes, MK11 3LW, UK
UKHW051940150726
7214IPUK00020B/357